S0-CBI-680

Lecture Notes in Biomathematics

91

Managing Editor:
S. A. Levin

Editorial Board:
Ch. DeLisi, M. Feldman, J. B. Keller, M. Kimura
R. May, J. D. Murray, G. F. Oster, A. S. Perelson
L. A. Segel

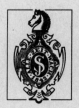

Frederik W. Wiegel

Physical Principles in Chemoreception

QP455
W54
1991

Springer-Verlag

Berlin Heidelberg New York
London Paris Tokyo
Hong Kong Barcelona
Budapest

Author

Frederik W. Wiegel
Center for Theoretical Physics
Department of Applied Physics
University of Twente
Enschede 7500 AE
The Netherlands

Mathematics Subject Classification (1991): 92C05, 92C45, 92E20

ISBN 3-540-54319-8 Springer-Verlag Berlin Heidelberg New York
ISBN 0-387-54319-8 Springer-Verlag New York Berlin Heidelberg

This work is subject to copyright. All rights are reserved, whether the whole or part of the material is concerned, specifically the rights of translation, reprinting, re-use of illustrations, recitation, broadcasting, reproduction on microfilms or in other ways, and storage in data banks. Duplication of this publication or parts thereof is only permitted under the provisions of the German Copyright Law of September 9, 1965, in its current version, and a copyright fee must always be paid. Violations fall under the prosecution act of the German Copyright Law.

© Springer-Verlag Berlin Heidelberg 1991
Printed in Germany

Typesetting: Camera ready by author
Printing and binding: Druckhaus Beltz, Hemsbach/Bergstr.
46/3140-543210 - Printed on acid-free paper

PREFACE

Is it not sheer foolishness to try to apply the methods of theoretical physics to biological structures? Physics flowered because it limited itself to the study of very simple systems; on the other hand, the essence of "living things" seems to have to do with the extreme intricacy of their structure. Is it a hopeless endeavour to attempt to bring the two together, or should one try nevertheless?

Most of my colleagues in theoretical physics feel one should not waste one's time and stick to "the good old hydrogen atom", but some of them feel one should try anyhow. This minority point of view was shared by Bohr in the thirties, Schrödinger in the fourties, Delbrück in the fifties and sixties, Purcell in the seventies, etc.

The theory of chemoreception represents only a very small part of this immense scientific question. Its study was started by Delbrück and others in the fifties. I was introduced to these problems by Charles DeLisi, during a visit to the National Institutes of Health in the summer of 1980. During the following decade I had the pleasure to collaborate with George Bell, Byron Goldstein, Alan Perelson and others at the Los Alamos National Laboratory. We studied a wide variety of questions, some of them relevant to the theory of chemoreception. I am grateful to them, both for the pleasure which our joint research always gives to me, as well as for their friendship and hospitality.

One of the pleasures of working in a university environment is the presence of intelligent young people who are still interested in learning something. I was lucky to have Bernard Geurts doing a Ph.D. dissertation on this topic. It is also a pleasure to teach a course on this subject, to the students in the Department of Applied Physics of Twente University. These students are in the third or fourth year of their engineering program. I teach this course two hours a week, for about ten weeks. The present monograph contains the lecture notes. I am indebted to Renate Maagdenberg for typing them with so much care.

These lecture notes do not claim to be the definitive treatise on the theory of chemoreception. If such a book can be written at all it should perhaps be done by Byron Goldstein, Carla Wofsy and others. I am looking forward to what the future might bring: comments of my readers, new theoretical concepts, more biological experiments.

Amsterdam   F.W.W.
Winter, 1990-1991

CONTENTS

I. GENERAL CONSIDERATIONS

1. Orders of magnitude and basic concepts

From the point of view of the physical sciences a living organism is a material system of staggering complexity. As a material object it must conform to all the laws of physics, yet its actual behaviour usually follows patterns which seem altogether alien to the world of physics. So, at the present stage of scientific sophistication one should study those living systems that are as simple as possible, and try to understand the physical principles which are involved in their behavior which is generally known as chemoreception (examples will be discussed shortly).

At this point in our discussion it is already instructive to make some rough order of magnitude estimates. Consider the "average" cell in the human body. This is of course not an actual cell which can be found somewhere in the reader's body, but it is a fictitious cell with properties which are the averages of the properties of the actual cells. These properties are listed in Table I.1; data partly taken from reference [1]. Comparing the mass of this cell with the typical mass of a human being one finds that the number of cells in the human body is of the order of magnitude 10^{14}. We shall used the symbol $\approx$ to indicate the order of magnitude of a quantity (that is: the value of this quantity apart from simple numerical factors like $\frac{4}{3}\pi$ or $\sqrt{3}$, so

$$\text{(number of cells in the human body)} \approx 10^{14}. \tag{1.1}$$

It is instructive to compare this with a typical astronomical number. For example, the number of stars in our galaxy is of the order of magnitude

$$\text{(number of stars in our galaxy)} \approx 10^{11}, \tag{1.2}$$

so the cells in the body are literally much more numerous than the stars in the sky. The number of cells in the nervous system, the weight of which is a few percent of the weight of the whole body, is given by the estimate

$$\text{(number of nerve cells)} \approx 10^{12} \text{ to } 10^{13}, \tag{1.3}$$

and a similare estimate holds for the number of cells in the immune system

$$\text{(number of cells of the immune system)} \approx 10^{12} \text{ to } 10^{13}. \tag{1.4}$$

When these numbers are compared to, for example the world's population, which is of the order 10^{10}, it becomes obvious that, in order for any living organism to function as a whole its cells must be involved in a continuous process of information exchange. Actually, most of the events in the life of a cell essentially involve physicochemical processes by which the cell detects the presence of certain chemical Table I.1 Properties of the average cell. Note the use of Ångstrom units (1 Å $= 10^{-10}$ m) and of micron units of length (1 $\mu = 10^{-6}$ m), which are customary in atomic physics c.q. cellular biology.

Shape   : Spherical
Radius   : 5×10^{-6} m $= 5 \times 10^4$ Å $= 5$ μ.
Volume   : 5.24×10^{-16} m^3
Density   : 1.03×10^3 kg m^{-3}
Mass   : 5.40×10^{-13} kg

compounds in its environment. The cell continuously monitors the presence of certain molecules which are either naturally present in its vicinity, or which have been emitted previously by other cells of the same or another organism. These chemical compounds (usually called ligands) are present in the extracellular medium in small concentrations, and move from cell to cell by means of Brownian motion, hydrodynamic convection, electromagnetic fields and other processes. A cell can detect those ligands which are important to its proper functioning by means of receptors. A receptor is a protein, or a complex consisting of proteins and other biopolymers, which somehow binds specifically with a certain ligand. Usually the receptors are embedded in the outher membrane of the cell. This means that there are as many receptor systems in the cell membrane as there are different types of ligands relevant to the cell's existence. Each receptor has a binding site which has the property that a ligand which is specific for this receptor is captured almost immediately, i.e. a ligand-receptor complex is formed almost immediately. Usually this complex acts in such a way that the ligand is rapidly transported through the membrane, which clears the receptor's binding site for its next catch. A nonspecific ligand will simply not react with the receptor. This process of a highly selective interaction of the cell with specific ligands is called chemoreception.

The present monograph is devoted to a discussion of the physical principles which are involved in various processes of chemoreception. In order to set the stage for the models and calculations of the following chapters we shall first discuss (i) the main protogonists in chemoreception; (ii) important examples of chemoreception and problems in the theory of chemoreception; (iii) chemoreception as a special example of that optimal use of physical laws by living things which has been noticed by many authors (most recently by Tributsch [2]).

2. Protagonists in chemoreception

(a) The cell is the smallest living thing, the basic structure of all plant and animal organization. It essentially consists of a mass of protoplasm, enclosed in a delicate membrane. The genetic material of the cell is usually packed in a central structure called the nucleus. Cells are of the most varied form and structure according to the functions which they have to perform, and any biomedical encyclopedia will list hunderds of different cell types [3]. For the purpose of quantitative descriptions one usually represents a cell by either one of the following three models:
(1) A sphere with a radius R which is typically given by $R = 5 \times 10^{-6}$ m, as indicated in Table I.1. This would be a rough model for a lymphocyte (white blood cell).

(2) A cylinder of radius R and height H. In the case where H >> R this would be a rough model for the axon of a nerve cell (cf. section 3(d)). For the erythrocyte (red blood cell), which is disk-shaped, the cylinder would also be an appropriate model, provided H < R.

(3) Some cells, for example the Purkinje cells in our nervous system, have an extremely complicated shape which resembles a tree with many branches, each of which branches again and again. Such cells should probably be described by the geometrical objects which are called fractals, and which have recently been studied especially by Mandelbrot [4]. To the author's knowledge very few actual calculations have yet been published in which cells are represented by fractals.

(b) The cell membrane. Research into the structure and function of the cell membrane (the delicate "skin" which shields the interior of the cell from its environment) has now reached such proportions that one can truly speak of the separate science of membranology, with its own specialized journals, textbooks, conferences and other modes of scientific communication. To the physicist the basic component of the cell membrane is a lipid membrane. In this subsection we shall briefly review the physics of the lipid bilayer; the biopolymers which are embedded in the bilayer form the subject of the next subsection.

There are many ways in which a physicist can look at a complicated object like a lipid bilayer. At the very detailed, molecular level of description he will represent the bilayer by two lipid monolayers which are apposed in such a way that the hydrophilic head groups of the lipids are in contact with the watery intra- and extracellular fluid, and the hydrophobic tails are shielded by the head groups from contact with water. The thickness h of this sandwich construction is typically of the order of magnitude

$$h \approx 50 \text{ Å} \tag{2.1}$$

At a much less detailed level of description the physicist will represent the lipid bilayer by a very thin sheet of continuous matter, embedded on both sides by water. In this macroscopic description the bilayer is fully characterized by a few macroscopic constants which will be discussed shortly.

The theoretical description of the lipid bilayer of course takes a very different form depending on the level of description which one uses. If one adopts the very detailed, molecular description the theory basically aims at actually calculating the movements of all parts of the many lipid molecules. Even for a very small part of a lipid monolayer this mechanistic approach leads to an extremely complicated calculational problem. Thanks to the availability of very fast electronic computing devices this numerical problem can actually be solved for very small model systems. For example Kox, Michels and Wiegel [5] showed in 1980 how one could use molecular dynamics to simulate a monolayer consisting of 90 "lipids", each consisting of a head group and a chain of six CH_2 groups. Similar molecular dynamics calculations for more refined models have also been performed by various groups, for example by Berendsen's group in Groningen [6]. One of the amusing features of these calculations is that, as the computer follows the movements of all molecules in the course of time, it can draw the actual configuration of the model lipid monolayer at some arbitrary time. For example, in the recent work of van Opheusden [7] one notices sizable fluctuations in head group spacings, which leads to the formation of pores, through which ions and small molecules might be able to diffuse across the membrane.

If, on the other hand, one uses the less detailed, macroscopic level of description the lipid bilayer becomes a thin sheet of continuous matter which is embedded on both sides in a watery continuum. In this case one is immediately faced with two questions: (1) What are the macroscopic constants which characterize this sheet of matter, for example, can you calculate them from a more microscopic model? (2) Given these macroscopic constants can you predict the relevant properties of the membrane; actually, what are the relevant properties and forms of behavior?

A considerable amount of research has been directed into attempts to calculate the macroscopic properties of the lipid bilayer from its microscopic structure. The general program of calculating the macroscopic properties of matter from its microscopic structure forms the topic of statistical physics, a venerable and sometimes frustrating part of theoretical physics, having its roots in the work of Boltzmann, Maxwell and Gibbs. In the context of membrane science one would hope that statistical physics could help us to predict the various phase transitions which occur in lipid membranes, elucidate the nature of the corresponding fluid- and solid phases, and help us to calculate the transport coefficients (like the viscosity and the elastic properties) of membranes. This has now been tried by many people, leading to an extensive theoretical literature which has partly been reviewed by Wiegel and Kox [8], Nagle [9] and Wiegel [11]. The fruits of this labor have been somewhat disappointing, mainly because of the very complicated nature of the many interactions between the various parts of the lipids and the watery substances outside of the membrane. For example, the theories do predict phase transitions to occur, but their precise locations are not predicted correctly; and the *a priori* calculations of, for example, the viscosity of a lipid bilayer seems almost hopelessly complicated.

Hence, at the time of writing it seems more feasible to assume some macroscopic model for the lipid membrane, for example a thin sheet of a viscous fluid, and to use its viscosity η' as an adjustable parameter (this membrane viscosity should of course not be confused with the ordinary viscosity η of the extracellular fluid). This phenomenological approach will often (but not always!) be used in the following pages. A phase transition in the membrane will now show up in a drastic change in the value of η', which will have considerable influence on the lateral diffusion of any object in the membrane, and thus on the efficiency of chemoreception.

(c) Membrane proteins. According to the fluid mosaic model of Singer and Nicolson [12] a biological membrane consists of a lipid bilayer in which a great variety of proteins are embedded. These proteins can cross-link to form complexes, and they can protrude on either or both sides of the membrane. As mentioned in section 1 a receptor molecule usually consists of a complex of such membrane proteins, often cross-linked with other biopolymers. For our theoretical studies we shall usually model the receptor molecule as a cylindrical disk with a height (h) equal to the thickness of the lipid bilayer and a radius (a) of about 100 Å. The binding site of the receptor is somewhat smaller and might be represented by a circular region of radius $s \approx 50$ Å.

The receptors (as well as all other membrane proteins) are subject to the Brownian movement, as a result of which they will diffuse laterally in the plane of the membrane. These diffusion processes will be discussed in detail in later chapters.

When a ligand binds to the binding site of a specific receptor the whole ligand-receptor complex can go through a configurational change, as a result of which the ligand is transported through the membrane and released into the interior of the cell. The precise nature of this configurational change is still unknown for most cases and forms the subject of vigorous biomedical research because of its enormous clinical significance. It seems likely that in some cases this configurational change is accompanied by conformational phase transitions akin to those which have been studied both experimentally and theoretically during the past 25 years (a review of the theoretical work is ref. [13]).

(d) The cytoskeleton. Once the ligand is released into the interior of the cell the subsequent events can develop along various lines. In many cases the ligand somehow interacts with the network of microtubules and microfilaments which lace the intracellular fluid and form the cytoskeleton. As a result the ligand is transported to one of the cell's organelles and stimulates (or inhibits) the cell's metabolism in a specific way, which was the goal of chemoreception to begin with.

At the time of writing structure and function of the cytoskeleton are still very poorly understood, as are many details of the functioning of the cell's genetic apparatus. Therefore, very few attempts have been made to model these processes yet (a notable exception is the work of the group of Blomberg, which is mainly concerned with kinetic aspects of the synthesis of biomolecules and with error correction in biosynthesis [14-23] and the work of Lindermann and Lauffenburger [48]). We shall shun this terra incognita in the following pages.

3. Examples of chemoreception

In this section several examples of chemoreception will be listed. We shall more or less follow the historical development of the various attempts at theoretical modeling, which is not the order in which these forms of chemoreception appeared in the course of phylogeny.

(a) Detection of pheromones. A pheromone is a substance which is secreted to the environment by an organism and perceived by a second organism of the same species, thereby producing a change in its behavior. A much-studied pheromone is the sex attractant *bombykol*, which is exuded in the air by the female silkworm moth *Bombyx mori*. So in this case the ligand is a bombykol molecule. The cell which is meant to detect the ligand is a sensory cell in the antennae system of the male of this species. This system was studied theoretically by Adam and Delbrück [24] and subsequently by Murray [25]. The study of Adam and Delbrück, which dates from the late sixties, is the first detailed model of chemoreception. It already contains some features of all later papers: their theory aims at calculating the number of ligands which are absorbed by the detecting cell per unit of time. They also recognize the possibility that chemoreception might occur in steps in which geometrical objects of decreasing dimensionality play a in steps in which geometrical objects of decreasing dimensionality play a role (multi-stage chemoreception with reduction of dimensionality; to be discussed later). Because of the roughly cylindrical shape of the sensory cell in Bombix mori refs. [24,25] use a cylindrical geometry rather than the spherical geometry which became fashionable later (cf. our discussion in section 2(a)).

(b) Chemotaxis. Next came the study of chemotaxis, which is the phenomenon that most unicellular microorganisms will move towards certain chemicals and away from others. Chemotaxis has been studied in much detail for the bacteria *Escherichia coli* and *Salmonella typhimurium* [26-31]. These bacteria execute a three-dimensional random walk: they swim steadily along a smooth trajectory (run), move briefly in a highly erratic manner (tumble), then run in a new direction [32,33]. They sense the local concentration of attractants or repellents and bias their random walk accordingly. For the spherical geometry which approximately describes these bacteria Berg and Purcell [34] developed a theory of the rate of capture of ligands by a large number of receptors which are distributed uniformly over the cell membrane. Ref. 34 is certainly the classical paper in this field, which has profoundly influenced all later authors. Two relevant monographs are by Koshland [45] and by Berg [46].

(c) The immune system. A third example of chemoreception, and probably the most important one, is the detection of antigens by the cells of the immune system. In this case the ligands are antigens, i.e. any microorganism, virus, cell, tissue or biopolymer which is foreign to the organism and which can induce a state of sensitivity of its immune system. The receptors are antibody molecules (immunoglobulins) embedded in the outer membrane of certain cells of the immune system.

The immune system forms the subject of a global, vigorous research effort, due to its crucial importance in our body's ability to keep itself alive and well. The total weight of all the cells which together form the immune system is roughly 5% of the total weight of the body, hence using the estimate (1.1) we found the estimate (1.4) for their number. These cells are literally scattered throughout the other cells, inspecting them while passing by. Somehow one class of cells in the immune system can tell whether a cell (or biopolymer, etc) belongs to the organism itself or if it is "foreign". If the cell is foreign it is killed by another group of cells of the immune system. In this way our bodies resemble the perfect totalitarian police state in which about 5% of the population constantly checks up on the other 95%!

The immune system is most remarkable in many respects. We list just a few of its exceptional features:

1. It can distinguish "self" from "foreign" with a very high accuracy.
2. It has a memory which relates to previous infections and diseases of the body. As a result of this memory:
3. It learns from its previous experiences by reacting more appropriately in the future.
4. It is the only organ which is present in (almost) every part of the body.
5. As a result of its omnipresence the immune system is also the most "holistic" part of the body, and the state of the immune system reflects the state of health of the individual with staggering finesse.

Immunology, the experimental study of the immune system, has now become a separate science which is accompanied by a huge literature. And the mathematical modeling of chemoreception by the immune system is also being developed in much detail, especially by groups at the Los Alamos National Laboratory and the National Institutes of Health. The interested reader is refered to monographs by DeLisi [35], Bell, Perelson and Pimbley [36], Perelson, DeLisi and Wiegel [10], and by Perelson [49] for reviews of the theoretical work.

(d) <u>Synaptic transmission</u>. Another example of chemoreception is the intermediate step in the transmission of a signal between two nerve cells. It is well known (cf., for example, Eccles [37]) that the process of synaptic transmission of a signal between two neurons involves essentially four stages:

(1) The signal (which is an electrochemical wave!) travels down to presynaptic axon and reaches the presynaptic knob. Here it somehow induces a change in the biochemical properties of the presynaptic membrane as a result of which a transmitter substance is secreted by the presynaptic cell.

(2) The molecules of the transmitter substance diffuse across the narrow synaptic cleft to the postsynaptic membrane where they are bound to specific receptors.

(3) The binding of transmitter molecules to receptors induces a change in the biochemical properties of the postsynaptic membrane in such a way that this membrane becomes selectively permeable to certain ions.

(4) The influx of these ions causes a change in the difference of the electric potential between the outside and the inside of the postsynaptic neuron. When this difference exceeds a certain treshold a new electrochemical wave originates in the vicinity of the postsynaptic membrane and travels down the postsynaptic axon.

It is of course step (2) in this sequence which involves the basic events of chemoreception. In this case the ligands are the molecules of the transmitter substance. There exist various transmitter substances: acetylcholine, glutamic acid, γ-aminobutyric acid and others. The nature of the receptor complex seems to be less well understood in this case than in the case of the immune response.

This form of chemoreception is essential for the proper functioning of our nervous system, and while reading this text billions of such events occur very second in your brain.

(e) <u>Olfaction and vision</u>. Chemoreception is essential, not only for the proper functioning of highly developed systems as the immune system or the nervous olfaction, which is the most important sense for many animals.

In man, of course, vision is usually felt to be the most important sense. From the point of view of the physics of chemoreception vision is unusual in several respects. First, the ligand is the photon, the quantum of light. A photon is an intrinsically quantum mechanical particle, and the astonishing fact that the capture of one or two single photons by a retinal cell can already lead to a subjective visual experience implies that our eyes are as sensitive to light as is compatible with the fundamental laws of nature!

Second, this peculiar form of chemoreception seems to be extremely old. Some bacteria already have a light-sensitive complex in their outer membrane, which they use to orient themselves with respect to the sun. It is believed that this sensitivity to light appeared in the primitive lifeforms on Earth about 3.7×10^9 years ago.

Third, the complicated biochemical events in photoreception in the vertebrate eye are relatively well understood. The retinal rod cell of the vertebrate eye is the favorite cell for many biochemical and biophysical studies of the phototransduction mechanism [38]. It turns out that, after a photon hits a rod cell, the process of phototransduction proceeds in three stages:

$$(\text{signal acquisition}) \rightarrow (\text{amplification}) \rightarrow (\text{expression}) \qquad (3.1)$$

Marc Bitenski [39] has called phototransduction the archetype of all the fundamental processes of life. One wonders if this is the reason why we identify so much with our visual representation of the world? Most of our concepts and symbols, both secular and spiritual, refer to the visual image of reality. It is actually very hard to understand what it "feels like" to be a creature for which a non-visual sense is the dominant one. This was, an effective communication with the dolphin, which experiences a world which is dominated by its highly developed senses of hearing and kinesthesia [40].

4. Problems in the theoretical physics of chemoreception

This monograph provides a manual for performing calculations on the diffusion of ligands in the vicinity of cells and on the rates of capture, escape or emission of ligands by cells. We shall successively discuss the following sequence of problems, starting with very simple ones and gradually progressing to the more complicate ones:

(a) The calculation of the translational diffusion coefficient of a ligand in the intercellular fluid.

(b) The calculation of the ligand current into a single receptor (the rate with which the receptor captures ligands). Here we shall first present some general results, next give details of the calculation for several models of the binding site, using a differential equation.

(c) For more complicated geometries of the binding site the differential equation approach is inappropriate because one cannot find an explicit solution. Instead, we develop complementary variational principles which enable one to find upper and lower bounds for the capture rate. Using these one can find approximate expressions for the capture rates of various complicated binding site geometries, and one can analyze the effect of receptor clustering.

(d) The calculation of the total ligand current into a cell of arbitrary shape, which carries a large number of receptors in its outer membrane. We shall include the possibility that there are forces acting between the ligands and the cell and that there is a flow field present too. The theory will be worked out especially for spherical cells and for cylindrical cells (cf. section 2(a)).

(e) Somewhat related to the previous subject is the calculation of the probabilities of capture and escape of a ligand by a single cell.

(f) Once the absorbing properties of a single cell are known one tends to ask more complicated questions. The first one is to calculate, for an arbitrary number of cells of arbitrary geometries (a "tissue" of absorbing cells), the mean time till ligand capture.

(g) Next we consider the capture of a large number of ligands by a tissue of absorbing cells, i.e. the decay of the total ligand population as a function of time. It will turn out that this decay often follows a non-exponential law, in contrast with what is usually assumed.

(h) As a preliminary to topics (i) and (j) we study lateral diffusion of a ligand immersed in the cell membrane, and we review various theoretical developments pertaining to this problem and to flow in the membrane.

(i) The diffusion of membrane protein is influenced considerably by their excluded volume; this will be the subject of detailed analysis.

(j) One now proceeds to the study of problems which have to do with two-stage chemoreception. In one-stage chemoreception the ligand can only be absorbed by the cell if it hits the binding site of a receptor molecule directly. In two-stage chemoreception the ligand is first incorporated in the cell membrane, and diffuses laterally in this membrane till it hits a binding site. In three-stage chemoreception the ligand first makes contact with the long biopolymers which are often attached to the outside of the cell membrane, diffuses along them to the membrane, next laterally in the membrane to a binding site.

(k) Other interesting problems have to do with hydrodynamic convection: the effect of the swimming of a cell on its rate of ligand capture; the effect of stirring of the surrounding fluid, etc.

(l) To close this list we should note the many open, unsolved problems which might be the subject of future research, and various more speculative comments which will be inserted in the text at the appropriate places.

5. Chemoreception and the optimal design of the cell

The study of chemoreception often leads to questions which have to do with the optimal design of the cell. This is a special case of the study of the shape and size of living things, which has fascinated many scientists from the days of D'Arcy Thompson [41] till the present time. Generally speaking the problem is to understand the shape and size of living creatures from the laws of physics and chemistry which hold for all matter, anywhere in the universe, animate or inanimate. We first discuss some simple examples, following a paper by Rau [42].

At the simplest level, where one only considers the static aspect of forms, much can be understood by using dimensional analysis. For a given group of life forms (for example land animals) of linear size L, surface and volume will be of the order of magnitude

$$\text{(surface)} \approx L^2$$

$$\text{(volume)} \approx L^3 \tag{5.1}$$

As the weight is proportional to the volume the bones of these animals must effectively support forces proportional to L^3. But the strength of a bone of thickness b is only proportional to b^2 and not to b^3. Hence one should expect that the thickness of the bones of most land animals will be proportional to

$$\text{(thickness of bones)} \sim L^{3/2} \tag{5.2}$$

where we use the symbol ~ to indicate proportionality. This obviously puts an upper limit on the size of a land animal and also explains why large animals tend to be clumsier than small animals: a bigger fraction of their volume is occupied by bones rather than muscles.

In water the force of gravity is more or less cancelled out by the buoyant force, so (5.2) is not true for sea animals. Also one should expect that the largest sea animals are much larger than the largest land animals (whales are large as compared to elephants).

Another application of this argument leads to the relation between the height of a tree and the diameter at its base

$$\text{(diameter at base)} \sim \text{(height of tree)}^{3/2} \, , \tag{5.3}$$

which turns out to be in good agreement with the sizes of actual trees.

Similar considerations play a role in the dynamics of living things. As an example we analyze walking. There is obviously an economy of effort if the legs swing at the rate of their natural angular frequency (ω), which is some function of the acceleration (g) of the Earth's gravitational field and the linear size (L) of the animal. So one puts

$$\omega \approx g^\alpha \, L^\beta \, , \tag{5.4}$$

where α and β are unknown exponents. Now the dimensions of these quantities are

$$[\omega] = [\, t \,]^{-1} \, , \tag{5.5a}$$

$$[g] = [\, \ell \,][\, t \,]^{-2} \, , \tag{5.5b}$$

$$[L] = [\, \ell \,] \, . \tag{5.5c}$$

If both sides of (5.4) are the same physical entity they must have the same dimension. Comparing the dimensions on both sides of (5.4) one finds from the powers of

$$\text{time } [t] \; : -1 = -2\alpha \, , \tag{5.6a}$$

$$\text{length } [\ell]: \; 0 = +\alpha + \beta \, . \tag{5.6b}$$

The solution is $\alpha = 1/2$, $\beta = -1/2$, so we have found the explicit formula

$$\omega = \text{(pure number)} \; g^{1/2} \, L^{-1/2} \, . \tag{5.7}$$

Here the "pure number" will be of order unity; you would have to know the precise shape of the leg to calculate it. But it is not interesting and the L-dependence of ω is given by

$$\omega \sim L^{-1/2} \, . \tag{5.8}$$

To length of the stride of an animal of size L will be proportional to L. So in walking the number of steps per unit of time is proportional to $L^{-1/2}$ whereas the length of each step is proportional to L. As a result one finds

$$\text{(speed)} \sim L^{1/2} \, . \tag{5.9}$$

This is called Froude's law, which turns out to hold for most land animals, as well as for fishes and birds.

Turning now to the cellular level one is immediately confronted with the remarkable fact that the cells of all organisms are roughly of the same size. For example, although an elephant is about 10^3 times the size of an ant (and 10^9 times its weight) the biological cells that constitute the elephant and the ant seldom show more than a factor 10 differences in size. This means that cells are optimal structures, which are used by nature as the building blocks for more complicated organisms.

At the time of writing there is no consensus about the sense in which the cell is an optimal structure, and which biophysical considerations are of fundamental importance in the design of this structure. Tentatively the following two global issues seem to be essential:

(a) *A proper balance between the consumption of energy and the capture of food.* The amount of energy needed by the cell, per unit of time, to stay alive and well will be proportional to its volume, so

$$\text{(rate of energy consumption)} \sim R^3 \ . \tag{5.10}$$

One should compare this with the rate at which the cell captures food. This is exactly one of the problems of chemoreception, specifically the problem discussed in section 4(d) for the case in which the ligands are food molecules, and most of this monograph is devoted to its solution. It will turn out that

$$\text{(rate of food intake)} \sim R \ . \tag{5.11}$$

Combination of the last estimates shows that the ratio

$$\frac{\text{food intake}}{\text{energy consumption}} \sim \frac{1}{R^2} \tag{5.12}$$

favors small cells, the smaller the better! But there is more to the life of a cell than just eating and drinking only; this brings us to the second global issue in its design.

(b) *Reliable storage of information.* A cell is also a depository of information, especially of the genetic information encoded in its DNA. One of the main functions of any cell is to act as a storage space for this information, i.e. the cell should provide a structure in which the genetic materials is sheltered safely from the Brownian movement and other dangers in its environment. This obviously favors large cells. The situation here is quite subtle because the information in the cell should be retrievable, which will only be the case if the cell is not too large.

It seems plausible to conjecture that the actual size and shape of the cell has arisen as the optimal solution to the competition between consideration (a) which favors small cells and (b) which favors large ones. Yet to the author's knowledge no quatitative models have been worked out; this remains as one of the major unsolved problems of theoretical biophysics.

Before we actually close this chapter we would like to draw the reader's attention to an important field of current scientific investigation, the only one that is truely interdisciplinary in the best sense of that word, and which is of relevance to the physics of chemoreception too. This is the work related to what is now generally called "the anthropic cosmological principle". For an introduction to the voluminous literature about this subject the reader is referred to the excellent textbooks by Davies [43] and by Barrow and Tipler [44]. In view of the existence of these recent monographs we can be rather short.

The anthropic cosmological principle arises when one studies the "design" of the Universe as a whole. One finds a hierarchy of structures and patterns. The largest structures have a size comparable to the radius of the Universe itself, a large but finite number which we shall estimate shortly. The smallest possible structures have a size which is often called Planck's length; this size too we shall estimate. This hierarchy of structures basically includes: the Universe itself, very large clusters of galaxies, smaller clusters of galaxies, clusters of stars, clouds of interstellar gas, stars and planetary systems, geophysical structures, meteorological structures, life-forms, molecules, atoms, atomic nuclei, protons and neutrons, maybe smaller elementary particles, Planck's length.

The second step towards the anthropic cosmological principle was taken by some scientists who noticed that this hierarchy of structures is essentially determined by the numerical values of the dimensionless constants of nature.

The third step consisted of three remarkable general features, which are supported by much experimental evidence:
(i) Dimensionless constants with a very different origin turn out to have the same order of magnitude.
(ii) These orders of magnitude are simple exponents of a number of the order 10^{+40}.
(iii) Organic life is possible because of these numerical coincidences.

There seems to be a principle at work here which cannot be formulated in a mathematical way but which can only be phrased verbally and somewhat vaguely: the anthropic cosmological principle. It says that the laws of physics (that is: the equations of physics, the numerical values of the dimensionless constants of nature which occur in these equations, and the initial conditions) must be such as to admit the existence of organic life and conscious observers at some stage. Using this principle one can derive many extremely unlikely coincidences between very different parts of physics, so the anthropic cosmological principle is far from a tautology.

Turning now to the problem of cellular design we would like to point to another remarkable coincidence. Suppose one would ask for the ideal intermediate scale of size, just in between the microcosm and the macrocosm. Calling this size x you want

$$\frac{x}{\text{Planck's length}} = \frac{\text{Radius of Universe}}{x} . \tag{5.13}$$

In order to calculate the numerical value of the solution

$$x = (\text{Planck's length})^{1/2} \ (\text{Radius of Universe})^{1/2} \tag{5.14}$$

we estimate the order of magnitude of the two quantities on the right hand side.

The radius of the Universe can be estimated with dimensional analysis in the following way. The general theory of relativity tells you that a space filled uniformly with matter will have a non-Euclidian geometry. The total volume will be finite, say of order R_0^3 where you could call R_0 the radius of the Universe. You know that R_0 can only be a function of:

c, the speed of light, because relativity is involved;

G, Newton's constant, because gravitation is involved;

ρ, the average mass density of the Universe.

Hence one puts

$$R_0 \approx c^\alpha G^\beta \rho^\gamma ,$$ (5.15)

where α, β and γ are unknown exponents. The dimensions are

$$[R_0] = [\ell] ,$$ (5.16a)

$$[c] = [\ell][t]^{-1} ,$$ (5.16b)

$$[G] = [\ell]^3 [m]^{-1} [t]^{-2} ,$$ (5.16c)

$$[\rho] = [m] [\ell]^{-3} .$$ (5.16d)

Comparing the dimensions on both sides of (5.15) one finds from the powers of

time [t] : $0 = -\alpha - 2\beta$, (5.17a)

length [ℓ]: $1 = \alpha + 3\beta - 3\gamma$, (5.17b)

mass [m] : $0 = -\beta + \gamma$. (5.17c)

The solution is $\alpha = 1$, $\beta = \gamma = -1/2$, so we have found the formula

$$R_0 = \text{(pure number)} \frac{c}{\sqrt{G\rho}} .$$ (5.18)

Here the "pure number" will be of order unity and can only be calculated using the whole formalism of the general theory of relativity. The value of this number is not interesting from our point of view because the order of magnitude of R_0 is given by the factor $\frac{c}{\sqrt{G\rho}}$.

Substituting the orders of magnitude $c \approx 10^8$ m sec^{-1}, $G \approx 10^{-10}$ m^3 kg^{-1} sec^{-2}, $\rho \approx 10^{28}$ kg m^{-3} one finds

$$R_0 \approx 10^{27} \text{ m} .$$ (5.19)

Next we estimate the order of magnitude of the smallest possible size, which is called Planck's length and usually denoted by L*. It is generally believed that such a smallest size exists because for objects with a size smaller than L* the quantum fluctuations of space itself would be too strong and destroy the object. The explicit value of L* should follow from a theory (which does not yet exist!) which combines the present theories of:

gravitation, which contains the constant G;

relativity, which contains the constant c;

quantum physics, which contains Planck's constant **h**.

Hence one puts

$$L^* = c^\alpha G^\beta h^\gamma .$$ (5.20)

As

$$[h] = [m][\ell]^2 [t]^{-1}$$ (5.21)

one finds

$$1 = \alpha + 3\beta + 2\gamma ,$$ (5.22a)

$$0 = -\alpha - 2\beta - \gamma ,$$ (5.22b)

$$0 = -\beta + \gamma .$$ (5.22c)

The solution is $\alpha = -3/2$, $\beta = \gamma = 1/2$, so one has found the formula

$$L^* = (\text{pure number}) \sqrt{\frac{G\hbar}{c^3}} .$$ (5.23)

Substituting $h \approx 10^{-35}$ kg m^2 sec^{-1} one finds the order of magnitude

$$L^* \approx 10^{-35} \text{ m} .$$ (5.24)

When the two estimates (5.19) and (5.24) are substituted into (5.14) the ideal intermediate scale of size x is found to be of order

$$x \approx 10^{-4} \text{ m} = 10^{+6} \text{ Å}$$ (5.25)

Referring to Table I.1 this is seen to be about 10 times the diameter of the average cell! So life at the cellular level seems to be a physical phenomenon that occurs on a scale of size which is ideally located between the microsm and the macrocosm; both the cause and the significance of this remarkable coincidence are at present unknown.

The interested reader might like to consult in this context also Delbrück's posthumous monograph [47].

References to chapter I

[1] P. Bongrand, C. Capo and R. Despieds. Physics of cell adhesion. Prog. Surface Sci. 12 (1982) 217-235.
[2] H. Tributsch. How life learned to live. MIT Press (Cambridge, Massachusetts, 1984).
[3] Stedman's medical dictionary. The Williams and Wilkins Company (Baltimore, 1976) 243-249.
[4] B.B. Mandelbrot. The fractal geometry of nature. Freeman and Company (San Francisco, 1982).
[5] A.J. Kox, J.P.J. Michels and F.W. Wiegel. Simulation of a lipid monolayer using molecular dynamics. Nature 287 (1980) 317-319.
[6] P. van der Ploeg and H.J.C. Berendsen. Molecular dynamics of a bilayer membrane. Mol. Physics 49 (1983) 233-248.
[7] J.H.J. van Opheusden. Theoretical studies of the lipid membrane and of macromolecules near a lipid membrane. Ph.D. Dissertation, Center for Theoretical Physics, Twente University of Technology (1987). Unpublished.
[8] F.W. Wiegel and A.J. Kox. Theories of lipid monolayers. Adv. Chem. Phys. 41 (1980) 195-228.

[9] J.F. Nagle. Theory of lipid bilayer phase transitions. Ann. Rev. Phys. Chem. 31 (1980) 157-199.

[10] A.S. Perelson, C. DeLisi and F.W. Wiegel Eds. Cell Surface Dynamics: Concepts and Models (Marcel Dekker Inc., New York, 1984).

[11] F.W. Wiegel. Ref 10 pg. 3-21.

[12] S.J. Singer and G.L. Nicolson. The fluid mosaic model of the structure of cell membranes. Science 175 (1972) 720-731.

[13] F.W. Wiegel. Conformational phase transitions and critical phenomena, Vol. 7. C. Domb and J.L. Lebowitz Eds. (Academic Press, London and New York, 1983) 100-149.

[14] C. Blomberg. A kinetic recognition process for t RNA at the ribosome. J. Theor. Biol. 66 (1977) 307-325.

[15] G. von Heijne, L. Nilsson and C. Blomberg. Translation and messenger RNA secondary structure. J. Theor. Biol. 68 (1977) 321-329.

[16] G. von Heijne, L. Nilsson and C. Blomberg. Models for m RNA translation: theory vs. experiment. Eur. J. Biochem. 92 (1978) 397-402.

[17] G. von Heijne and C. Blomberg. The concentration dependence of the error frequencies and some related quantities in protein synthesis. J. Theor. Biol. 78 (1979) 113-120.

[18] M. Ehrenberg and C. Blomberg. Thermodynamic constraints on kinetic proofreading in biosynthetic pathways. Biophys. J. 31 (1980) 333-358.

[19] C. Blomberg, M. Ehrenberg and C.G. Kurland. Free-energy dissipation constraints on the accuracy of enzymatic selection. Quart. Rev. Biophys. 13 (1980) 231-254.

[20] C. Blomberg and M. Ehrenberg. Energy considerations for kinetic proofreading in biosynthesis. J. Theor. Biol. 88 (1981) 631-670.

[21] C. Blomberg, M. Ehrenberg and C.G. Kurland. Free-energy driven error correction in macromolecular biosynthesis: a theoretical approach. Acta Chem. Scand. B35 (1981) 223-224.

[22] C. Blomberg. Thermodynamic aspects of accuracy in the synthesis of biomolecules. Int. J. Quant. Chem. 23 (1983) 687-707.

[23] C. Blomberg. Free-energy cost and accuracy in branched selection processes of biosynthesis. Quart. Rev. Biophys. 16 (1983) 415-519.

[24] G. Adam and M. Delbrück. Reduction of dimensionality in biological diffusion processes. In: Structural Chemistry and Molecular Biology, Eds. A. Rich and N. Davidson (W.H. Freeman and Company, San Francisco, 1968) 198-215.

[25] J.D. Murray. Lectures on Nonlinear-Differential-Equation Models in Biology (Clarendon Press, Oxford, 1977) 83-127.

[26] J. Adler. Chemoreceptors in bacteria. Science 166 (1975) 1588-1597.

[27] J. Adler. Chemotaxis in bacteria. Ann. Rev. Biochem. 44 (1975) 341-356.

[28] H.C. Berg. Bacterial behavior. Nature 254 (1975) 389-392.

[29] H.C. Berg. Chemotaxis in bacteria. Ann. Rev. Biophys. Bioeng. 4 (1975) 119-136.

[30] H.C. Berg. How bacteria swim. Sci. Am. 233 (2) (1975) 36-44.

[31] J. Adler. The sensing of chemicals by bacteria. Sci. Am. 234 (4) (1976) 40-47.

[32] H.C. Berg and D.A. Brown. Chemotaxis in Escherichia coli analysed by three-dimensional tracking. Nature 239 (1972) 500-504.

[33] H.C. Berg and L. Turner. Movements of microorganisms in viscous enviroments. Nature 278 (1979) 349-351.

[34] H.C. Berg and E.M. Purcell. Physics of chemoreception. Biophys. J. 20 (1977) 193-219.

[35] G. DeLisi. Antigen-Antibody Interactions (Springer Verlag, New York, 1976).

[36] G.I. Bell, A.S. Perelson and G.H. Pimbley. Theoretical Immunology (Marcel Dekker Inc., New York, 1978)

[37] J.C. Eccles. The Understanding of the Brain (McGraw-Hill, New York, 1973).

[38] M. Chabre. Trigger and amplification mechanisms in visual phototransduction. Ann. Rev. Biophys. Chem. 14 (1985) 331-360.

[39] M. Bitenski, private communication.

[40] J.C. Lilly. Lilly on Dolphins (Anchor Press, Garden City, 1975).

[41] D'Arcy W. Thompson. On Growth and Form (Cambridge University Press, Cambridge, 1917, reprinted in 1943).

[42] A.R.P. Rau. Of shapes and sizes. Sc. Today, Oct. (1977) 15-20.

[43] P.C.W. Davies. The Accidental Universe (Cambridge University Press, Cambridge, 1982).

[44] J.D. Barrow and F.J. Tipler. The anthropic Cosmological Principle (Oxford University Press, Oxford, 1986).

[45] D.E. Koshland. Bacterial Chemotaxis as a Model Behavioral System (Raven Press, New York, 1980).

[46] H.C. Berg. Random Walks in Biology (Princeton University Press, Princeton, 1983).

[47] M. Delbrück. Mind from Matter? (Blackwell, Palo Alto, 1986).

[48] J.J. Linderman and D.A. Lauffenburger. Receptor/Ligand Sorting along the Endocytic Pathway (Springer, New York, 1989) Lecture Notes in Biomathematics 78.
[49] A.S. Perelson Ed. Theoretical Immunology Vols. I and II (Addison-Wesley, Reading CA, 1988).

Short list of symbols used in chapter I

a   Radius of the circular region which represents the binding site on a receptor complex

c   speed of light

η Viscosity of the extracellular fluid

η' Viscosity of the lipid membrane

G   Newton's constant

h   Thickness of the lipid bilayer. Not to be confused with Planck's constant, which only plays a role in section I.5

h   Planck's constant, only in section I.5

H   Heigth of a cylindrical cell

L*   Planck's length

R   Radius of a spherical cell or radius of a cylindrical cell

R_0 Radius of the Universe

s   Radius of the circular region which represents the binding site on a receptor complex

$\approx$ Order of magnitude

$\sim$ proportionality

$=$ equality

$\cong$ approximate equality

II. SPATIAL DIFFUSION

1. The translational- and rotational diffusion coefficients

The calculation of the translational diffusion coefficient D_T of proteins and other ligands in the intercellular fluid forms the subject of a vast literature; some of the classical papers are those by Chandrasekhar [1] and Einstein [2]. This transport coefficient is defined by the relation

$$\vec{j} = -D_T \, \vec{\nabla} c \, , \tag{1.1}$$

where $c(\vec{r},t)$ denotes the number density of ligands and $\vec{j}(\vec{r},t)$ their current density. In the papers just quoted it is shown from the general principles of statistical physics that the diffusion coefficient is related to the translational friction coefficient f_T by the Einstein relation

$$f_T D_T = k_B T \, , \tag{1.2}$$

where k_B denotes Boltzmann's constant and T the absolute temperature. This enables one to determine D_T from a calculation of f_T, which is defined as the hydrodynamic drag force on the ligand, per unit relative velocity.

For many models of the ligand the friction coefficient can be calculated *a priori*. Consider, for example, the case in which the ligand is represented by a small hard sphere of radius a and the extracellular fluid by a Newtonian fluid of viscosity η and mass density ρ_0. Let the sphere be fixed at the origin of a Cartesian set of coordinates and let the asymptotic fluid velocity be directed along the negative z-axis with velocity v_0. One has to solve the pressure $P(\vec{r},t)$ and velocity $\vec{v}(\vec{r},t)$ from the Navier-Stokes equation and the continuity equation for an incompressible fluid

$$\rho_0 \left(\tfrac{\partial}{\partial t} + \vec{v} \cdot \vec{\nabla} \right) \vec{v} = -\vec{\nabla} P + \eta \Delta \vec{v} \, , \tag{1.3a}$$

$$\operatorname{div} \vec{v} = 0 \, , \tag{1.3b}$$

subject to the boundary conditions that $\vec{v}$ tends to a vector with components $(0,0,-v_0)$ at large distances from the sphere, and that $\vec{v} = \vec{0}$ at the surface of the sphere. The latter "stick" boundary condition is sometimes replaced by the "slip" boundary condition that $\vec{v}$ should be parallel to the surface of the sphere. For a time-independent flow problem the term $\partial \vec{v}/\partial t$ in (1.3) can be omitted.

The ratio of the orders of magnitude of the non-linear term to the term $\eta \, \Delta \, \vec{v}$ is given by the Reynolds number

$$\mathbb{R} \equiv \frac{a \, v_0 \, \rho_0}{\eta} \, . \tag{1.4}$$

For a ligand with mass m the average kinetic energy is $\tfrac{3}{2} k_B T$ so

$$v_0 \approx (k_B T/m)^{1/2} . \tag{1.5}$$

Hence the Reynolds number has the order of magnitude

$$\mathbb{R} \approx \frac{a\rho_0}{\eta} \left(\frac{k_B T}{m} \right)^{1/2} , \tag{1.6}$$

and with the typical values $a \approx 2 \times 10^{-7}$ cm, $\eta \approx 10^{-2}$ g cm^{-1} s^{-1}, $\rho_0 = 1$ g cm^{-3}, $k_B T \approx 4 \times 10^{14}$ cm^2 g s^{-2} and m $\approx 10^{17}$ g one finds $\mathbb{R} \approx 10^3$. Hence one can replace the Navier-Stokes equation by its linearized form

$$-\vec{\nabla}P + \eta\Delta\vec{v} = 0 \tag{1.7}$$

to a very good approximation. The solution of this equation with stick boundary conditions can be found, for example, in the monograph of Landau and Lifshitz [3]. In spherical coordinates (r,ϕ,θ) the velocity components in the direction of increasing values of r and θ are given by

$$v_r = -v_0 \cos \theta \left[1 - \frac{3a}{2r} + \frac{a^3}{2r^3} \right] , \tag{1.8}$$

$$v_\theta = +v_0 \sin \theta \left[1 - \frac{3a}{4r} - \frac{a^3}{4r^3} \right] . \tag{1.9}$$

From this flow field the pressure and the viscous force exerted on the sphere can be calculated; this leads to the Stokes formula for the drag force (F) on the sphere

$$F = 6 \pi \eta a v_0 . \tag{1.10}$$

Hence the friction coefficient is given by

$$f_T = \frac{F}{v_0} = 6 \pi \eta a , \tag{1.11}$$

and the diffusion coefficient by

$$D_T = \frac{k_B T}{6 \pi \eta a} . \tag{1.12}$$

Using the orders of magnitude just quoted one finds values for the translational diffusion coefficient, at physiological temperatures, which are of the order 10^{-6} cm^2 s^{-1}, in agreement with the experiments.

Further corrections to the Stokes approximation, due to the non-linear term in the Navier-Stokes equation, have been discussed by several authors (cf. van Dyke [4]). For example, the right-hand side of (1.10) turns out to be the first term of an asymptotic expansion in the Reynolds number

$$F = 6 \pi \eta a v_0 \left\{ 1 + \frac{3}{8} \mathbb{R} + \frac{9}{40} \mathbb{R}^2 \, \ell n \, \mathbb{R} + 0(\mathbb{R}^2) \right\} . \tag{1.13}$$

Hence for the small Reynolds numbers found in chemoreception the expression (1.12) should be an excellent approximation.

For the sake of completeness we also note the expression for the rotational diffusion coefficient (D_R) of a protein immersed in a Newtonian fluid. For the hard sphere model one finds (cf. ref. [5])

$$D_R = \frac{k_B T}{8 \pi \eta a^3} . \tag{1.14}$$

It is perhaps of some use to the reader to point out that the general form of the expressions (1.12) and (1.14) already follows from dimensional analysis. In order to demonstrate this for eq. (1.12) one notices that use of the linearized form (1.7) of the Navier-Stokes equation leads to a linear relation between the drag force F and the velocity of the sphere v_0. As the only other parameters are η and a one must have a relation of the form

$$F \approx v_0 \, \eta^\alpha \, a^\beta .$$

The dimensions are $[F] = [m] \, [\ell] \, [t]^{-2}$, $[v_0] = [\ell] \, [t]^{-1}$, $[\eta] = [m] \, [\ell]^{-1} \, [t]^{-1}$ and $[a] = [\ell]$. Hence one equates the powers of

mass : $1 = \alpha$,
length: $1 = 1 - \alpha + \beta$,
time : $-2 = -1 - \alpha$,

which set of equations has the unique solution $\alpha = \beta = 1$, leading to the formula $F \approx \eta \, a \, v_0$ and hence to $D_T \approx k_B T / \eta a$. In a similar way one finds for the rotational diffusion coefficient $D_R \approx k_B T / \eta a^3$.

The *a priori* determination of the translational- and rotational diffusion coefficients is also possible for non-spherical shapes of the ligand and for ligands that are permeable polymer coils or porous complexes of crosslinked macromolecules. These calculations are the subject of a small monograph [5] to which the reader is refered for all derivations. In [5] it was pointed out that for a protein the impermeable sphere model (for which 1.12 and 1.14 hold) can be somewhat unrealistic because a large protein in solution often has a rather open, random coil configuration. As a result, the fluid can flow through as well as around the protein and one is faced with the problem of finding a theoretical description for flow through a porous macromolecular system.

The most convenient way to characterize a porous macromolecular coil is by means of a new material constant, the hydrodynamic permeability k, which has the dimension of $[\text{length}]^2$ and which can either be constant throughout the coil or a function of the radial distance to the center of the coil. In the case of a homogeneous porous medium the physical meaning of k can be visualized by the following fictitious experiment. Consider a half-space filled with this porous medium, and a fluid that permeates it, and which flows with a constant velocity v_0 (parallel to the fluid-medium boundary) in the other half-space outside the porous medium. Inside the porous medium the fluid velocity will be parallel to the boundary and its magnitude will decrease according to the formula

$$v(x) = v_0 \exp \left(- \frac{x}{\sqrt{k}} \right) , \tag{1.15}$$

where x denotes the distance from a point inside the porous medium to the boundary. This result shows that the quantity $\sqrt{k}$, which has the dimension of a length, is a rough measure for the distance by which flow outside a porous medium effectively penetrates into the medium. For that reason $\sqrt{k}$ is sometimes called the penetration depth. In typical polymer-solvent mixtures $\sqrt{k}$ is of the order of 10 to 10^2 Å.

The translational and rotational diffusion coefficients have been calculated for several models of permeable polymer coils, as reviewed in [5]. For example, if the permeability is a constant (k_0) throughout the volume of the coil, the flow pattern and all other physical quantities are determined by the value of the dimensionless quantity

$$\sigma = \frac{a}{\sqrt{k_0}} . \tag{1.16}$$

The diffusion constants are found to be given by

$$D_T = \frac{k_B T}{6 \pi \eta \alpha} \left[\frac{3}{2\sigma^2} + \frac{1}{G_0(\sigma)} \right] ; \quad G_0(\sigma) \equiv 1 - \frac{1}{\sigma} \frac{e^\sigma - e^{-\sigma}}{e^\sigma + e^{-\sigma}} , \tag{1.17}$$

$$D_R = \frac{k_B T}{8 \pi \eta a^3} \left[1 + \frac{3}{\sigma^2} - \frac{3}{\sigma} \frac{e^\sigma + e^{-\sigma}}{e^\sigma - e^{-\sigma}} \right]^{-1} . \tag{1.18}$$

A more realistic model would be characterized by a low permeability near the center of the coil and high permeability near the fringes. For such a model (the Gaussian coil) accurate numerical results can be found in [5].

2. General comments on diffusion

The diffusion of ligands is a special case of the random walks which often occur in biology (a recent monograph by H.C. Berg is exclusively devoted to them [6]). The value $D_T \approx 10^{-6}$ cm^2 s^{-1} for the translational diffusion coefficient of a typical ligand sets the scale for several physiological relaxation processes which are dominated by diffusion. For example, the average square of the distance over which a ligand travels in time t equals

$$\langle \vec{r}^2 \rangle = 6 D_T t \tag{2.1}$$

in three dimensions. As the diameter of a cell is typically of order $2R \approx 10^{-3}$ cm (Table I.1) the time which a ligand needs to diffuse over a distance comparable to the cell diameter is of the order 0.16 s. When two cell membranes are apposed their distance is of order 10^2 Å $= 10^{-6}$ cm. In this case - which applies to the synaptic transmission of a signal between two neurons - the transmitter substance needs as little as 5×10^{-7} s to diffuse across the synaptic cleft between the nerve cells. These time scales are typical for various physiological processes.

It is perhaps also of some interest to mention the most peculiar shape of the actual trajectory of a diffusing particle. These trajectories are highly irregular when studied on any scale of coarse graining in space and time. Another way to phrase this is by imagining a series of microscopes with increasing resolving power. The irregularities seen at one magnification turn out to contain finer irregularities at a higher magnification; when these are magnified they show even finer irregularities, and so on. The trajectories of diffusing ligands are fractals in the mathematical sense (cf. section I.2 (a) 3). They are discussed by Mandelbrot in ref. I-4 as well as in an older monograph [7].

Of course, the description of the trajectory of a physical object (the ligand) by a mathematical entity like a fractal has its limit of validity. In the case under consideration this limit appears when the trajectory is followed on a time scale small compared to the time t_0 between two successive collisions between the ligand and particles from the solvent (H_2O molecules). The time t_0 defines the smallest time scale in the hierarchy of diffusional time scales in biophysics; its magnitude can be estimated as follows. A solvent particle with mass m and momentum p will have an average kinetic energy $<p^2/2m> = (3/2)k_BT$. Hence the absolute value Δp of the momentum transfer in each collision between a solvent particle and the ligand under consideration will be of the order of magnitude

$$\Delta p \approx \sqrt{mk_BT} \ . \tag{2.2}$$

If there are ω such collisions per second the total magnitude of the force will be of order $\omega\Delta p$. But this equals $4\pi a^2 P$, where a denotes the radius of the ligand, visualized as a sphere, and P the pressure. Hence the number of collisions per second is of order

$$\omega \approx \frac{4\pi a^2 P}{\Delta p} \ . \tag{2.3}$$

Substituting $a \approx 20$ Å, $P = 1$ atm $\cong 10^6$ dyn cm^{-2}, $k_BT \approx 4 \times 10^{14}$ cm^2 g s^{-2} and $m \approx 10^{22}$ g in the last two equations, one finds $\omega \approx 2.4 \times 10^{11}$ s^{-1}. This implies that $t_0 \approx 0.4 \times 10^{11}$ s. The trajectory of the ligand will consist of a straight line between successive collisions with solvent molecules; that is, when the trajectories of the diffusing particles are studied on time scales $\leq t_0$, they are smooth and no "fractal behavior" will be seen.

3. The effects of excluded volume on the thermal equilibrium distribution of ligands

When the ligand concentration becomes high the steric interactions between the ligands might become important. In two recent papers Goldstein and the author studied the effects of excluded volume on the distribution of ligands, both in equilibrium and in stationary non-equilibrium situations [8,9]. In this section we shall briefly discuss the effects of excluded volume on the equilibrium distribution of ligands, using the methods of equilibrium statistical mechanics. First we discuss the case in which there is only one type of ligand, next we consider the case in which there are two types of ligands.

Suppose N ligands are distributed over some part of space. Their only interactions are steric repulsions, such that in the close-packed configuration each ligand blocks a volume equal to a^3. In general N will be smaller than the number of ligands needed for close-packing so $Na^3 <$ total volume available. In order to characterize a macroscopic distribution we divide the total available volume (which may have any shape) into a set of small regions. The size of a region must be small as compared to the size of the volume; hence the energy of a ligand in region i is practically constant within the region; call it E_i. Moreover, the linear size of a region must be large as compared to a; hence the maximum number of ligands which can be packed into region i is large as compared to unity (call this number g_i).

A distribution of the ligands is a sequence of numbers $\{n_i\}$ where n_i equals the number of ligands inside region i. The total statistical weight $W\{n_i\}$ which has to be assigned to a particular distribution $\{n_i\}$ is the product of the following three factors:

(i) A factor

$$\frac{N!}{\prod_i n_i!} \qquad (3.1)$$

equal to the number of ways to divide N distinguishable ligands into clusters of n_i.

(ii) For each region a factor

$$g_i (g_i-1) \, ... \, (g_i-n_i+1) = \frac{g_i!}{(g_i-n_i)!} \qquad (3.2)$$

equal to the number of ways to divide the n_i distinguishable ligands in region i over the g_i possible sites in that region.

(iii) A Boltzmann factor

$$\exp(-\beta\Sigma_i n_i E_i), \qquad (3.3)$$

where $\beta = (k_B T)^{-1}$.

Collecting these results one finds that the *a priori* statistical weight of the distribution $\{n_i\}$ equals

$$W\{n_i\} = N! \exp(-\beta \sum_i n_i E_i) \prod_i \frac{g_i!}{n_i! \, (g_i-n_i)!} \, . \qquad (3.4)$$

We now identify the thermal equilibrium distribution $\{n_i^*\}$ with that distribution for which W is as large as possible, subject to the constraint

$$\sum_i n_i = N \qquad (3.5)$$

that the total number of ligands is constant. Introducing a Lagrange multiplier μ it can be shown that the equilibrium distribution can be solved from the relation

$$\frac{\partial}{\partial n_i} (\ell n \, W + \mu \sum_j n_j) = 0 \qquad (3.6)$$

without condition (3.5), provided μ is choosen afterwards in such a way that (3.5) is satisfied. As all quantities g_i and n_i are large as compared to unity one can use Stirlings approximation

$$\ell n \, x! \cong x \, \ell n \, x - x \, , \qquad (x \gg 1) \qquad (3.7)$$

to calculate $\ell n \, W$. One finds in a straightforward way

$$\frac{n_i^*}{g_i} = \frac{1}{1 + e^{\beta E_i - \mu}} \tag{3.8}$$

for the equilibrium distribution of the ligands over the available part of space.

Before we consider the case of two types of proteins a few comments are in order:

(a) As remarked before, the constant μ must be calculated from

$$\sum_i \frac{g_i}{1 + e^{\beta E_i - \mu}} = N. \tag{3.9}$$

(b) The result (3.8), which was found previously by Ryan et al. [10], shows a formal similarity with the Fermi-Dirac distribution. This similarity is fortuitous as the ligands can be treated as distinguishable, classical particles rather than as fermions which are indistinguishable quantum particles.

(c) If the ligands are described by a local number density $c(\vec{r},t)$, as has to be done in a diffusion-equation approach, the relation between their equilibrium density $c(\vec{r},\infty)$ and n_i^* is given by

$$c(\vec{r}_i,\infty) = \frac{n_i^*}{a^3 g_i} = a^{-3} \left[1 + e^{\beta E_i - \mu} \right]^{-1}, \tag{3.10}$$

where $\vec{r}_i$ is at the position of region i. This shows that μ will be independent of g_i.

Now consider the case in which there are two types of ligand, say N' of type 1 and N'' of type 2. It is straightforward to generalize the preceeding theory to this case, provided both types of ligand block the same effective volume a^3. A distribution is now a sequence of numbers $\{n_i', n_i''\}$ where n_i' equals the number of type 1 ligands in region i, and n_i'' the number of type 2 ligands. Let the energies in region i be E_i' and E_i''. The relevant combinatorial weight factors (3.1 - 3) now become

(i) $$\left[\frac{N'!}{\prod_i n_i'!} \right] \left[\frac{N''!}{\prod_i n_i''!} \right], \tag{3.11}$$

(ii) $$\frac{g_i!}{(g_i - (n_i' + n_i''))!}, \tag{3.12}$$

(iii) $$\exp \left\{ -\beta \sum_i (n_i' E_i' + n_i'' E_i'') \right\} \tag{3.13}$$

respectively. Hence the weight of a distribution is

$$W\{n_i', n_i''\} = N'! N''! \exp\{-\beta \sum_i (n_i' E_i' + n_i'' E_i'')\} \prod_i \frac{g_i!}{n_i'! n_i''! (g_i - n_i' - n_i'')!}. \tag{3.14}$$

There are two Lagrange multipliers μ' and μ'' to take into account the two constraints

$$\sum_i n_i' = N' \quad , \quad \sum_i n_i'' = N'' . \tag{3.15a,b}$$

The thermal equilibrium distribution $\{n_i'^*, n_i''^*\}$ must now be solved from the two relations

$$\frac{\partial}{\partial n_i'} (\ell n\ W + \mu' \sum_i n_i' + \mu'' \sum_i n_i'') = 0 \ , \tag{3.16}$$

$$\frac{\partial}{\partial n_i''} (\ell n\ W + \mu' \sum_i n_i' + \mu'' \sum_i n_i'') = 0 \ . \tag{3.17}$$

Using Stirling's approximation one easily finds the solution

$$\frac{n_i'^*}{g_i} = \frac{1}{1 + e^{\beta E_i' - \mu'} + e^{\beta E_i' - \beta E_i'' - \mu' + \mu''}} \ , \tag{3.18}$$

$$\frac{n_i''^*}{g_i} = \frac{1}{1 + e^{\beta E_i'' - \mu''} + e^{\beta E_i'' - \beta E_i' - \mu'' + \mu'}} \tag{3.19}$$

for the thermal equilibrium distribution of the two types of ligand through the available part of space. Note that their ratio is

$$\frac{n_i'^*}{n_i''^*} = e^{\beta(E_i'' - E_i') + \mu' - \mu''} \ . \tag{3.20}$$

The two constants μ' and μ'' must be picked in such a way that eqs. (3.15a,b) are satisfied.

References to chapter II

[1] S. Chandrasekhar. Stochastic problems in physics and astronomy. Rev. Mod. Phys. 15 (1943) 1-89. Reprinted in: Selected papers on noise and stochastic processes, ed. N. Wax (Dover, New York, 1954).
[2] A. Einstein. Investigations on the theory of the Brownian movement (Dover, New York, 1956).
[3] L.D. Landau and E.M. Lifshitz. Fluid Mechanics (Pergamon, London, 1959) §20.
[4] M. van Dyke. Perturbation Methods in Fluid Mechanics (Parabolic Press, Stanford, 1975).
[5] F.W. Wiegel. Fluid Flow through Porous Macromolecular Systems. Lecture Notes in Physics 121 (Springer, Heidelberg, 1980).
[6] H.C. Berg. Random Walks in Biology. (Princeton University Press, Princeton, 1983).
[7] B.B. Mandelbrot. Fractals (Freeman, San Francisco, 1977).
[8] B. Goldstein and F.W. Wiegel. The effects of excluded volume on the equilibrium distribution of cell membrane proteins. Preprint (1990).
[9] F.W. Wiegel and B. Goldstein. Kinetics of diffusing membrane proteins: excluded volume effects. Preprint (1990).
[10] T.A. Ryan, J. Myers, D. Holowka, B. Baird and W.W. Webb. Science 239 (1988) 61.

III. LIGAND CURRENT INTO A SINGLE RECEPTOR

1. General considerations and dimensional analysis

If no ligands are created or annihalated in the intercellular medium ligand conservation is expressed by the equation

$$\frac{\partial c}{\partial t} = - \text{div } \vec{j} .$$

(1.1)

In the simplest case, in which there are no external forces or convective fluid motions, combination with II.1.1 gives the diffusion equation

$$\frac{\partial c}{\partial t} = D_T \Delta c .$$

(1.2)

In this chapter we shall calculate the ligand current into a single receptor, if the ligand concentration equals $c(\infty)$ far from the receptor. This means that the time-dependent equation

$$\Delta c = 0$$

(1.3)

has to be solved under the following boundary conditions: (a) At large distances from the receptor

$$c \to c(\infty) .$$

(1.4a)

(b) The binding site is a perfect absorber, hence

$$c = 0$$

(1.4b)

at the surface of the binding site. (c) The rest of the cell membrane is a reflector of ligands. As the size of the binding site is very small as compared to the size of the cell the shape of the cell surface in the vicinity of the binding site is often assumed to be flat. In a Cartesian set of coordinates with the x,y plane coinciding with the surface of the cell membrane this implies

$$\frac{\partial c}{\partial z} = 0, \qquad\qquad (z = 0),$$

(1.5)

outside of the binding site.

Once this problem is solved the total ligand current into the receptor site is given by the surface integral

$$J = - \oint \vec{j} \cdot d^2\vec{S}$$

(1.6)

where $d^2\vec{S}$ is directed into the extracellular medium. From (1.3), (II.1.1) and boundary condition (a) it is clear that the ligand current density has the form $\vec{j} = D_T c(\infty)\vec{j}'$, where $\vec{j}'$ depends on the binding site, but not on D_T or $c(\infty)$. This implies that the ligand current has the form $J = D_T c(\infty)J'$, where J' does not depend on D_T or $c(\infty)$. Comparing dimensions on both sides one finds that the dimension of J' equals $[J'] = [\text{length}]$. Hence, if the linear dimensions of the binding site can be characterized by a single length s the current J' must be proportional to s and

$$J = \alpha \, D_T c(\infty)s, \tag{1.7}$$

where the value of the numerical constant α depends on the geometrical shape of the binding site, but not on its size, nor on D_T or $c(\infty)$. As the geometrical shape of the binding sites of most chemoreceptors is unknown it is of some interest to calculate the constant α for various models; this is the subject of the following sections.

2. Hemispherical binding site

Suppose the binding site is a hemisphere of radius s with the equatorial plane coinciding with the surface of the cell membrane. In this case one has to find the spherically symmetric solution of (1.3), which now reads in spherical coordinates (r,θ,ϕ)

$$\left(\frac{d^2}{dr^2} + \frac{2}{r} \frac{d}{dr} \right) c(r) = 0. \tag{2.1}$$

The boundary conditions are

$$c(s) = 0, \qquad c \to c(\infty) \quad \text{for} \quad r \to \infty . \tag{2.2}$$

The reflecting wall boundary condition (1.5) in the equatorial plane outside the binding site is satisfied automatically because of the spherical symmetry of the solution

$$c(r) = c(\infty) \left(1 - \frac{s}{r} \right) , \qquad (r \geq s) . \tag{2.3}$$

The magnitude of the ligand current density at the surface of the binding site is

$$j = D_T \left[\frac{dc}{dr} \right]_{r=s} = D_T c(\infty)/s. \tag{2.4}$$

As the area of the binding site is $2\pi s^2$ the ligand current is

$$J = 2\pi D_T c(\infty)s, \tag{2.5}$$

which corresponds to (1.7) with $\alpha = 2\pi$. Note that (2.3) implies that the perturbation of the uniform concentration, due to capture of ligands, extends over a distance of order of magnitude s.

3. Plane circular binding site

Another possible geometry of the binding site is a circular region of radius s in the plane of the membrane. In this case it seems natural to transform (1.3) to cylindrical coordinates (r,ϕ,z) where $z = 0$ corresponds to the cell membrane. As the stationary state can be expected to have cylindrical symmetry one finds

$$\left[\frac{\partial^2}{\partial r^2} + \frac{1}{r} \frac{\partial}{\partial r} + \frac{\partial^2}{\partial z^2} \right] c(r,z) = 0 \qquad (z \geq 0), \tag{3.1}$$

with the boundary conditions

$$c \to c(\infty) \quad \text{for} \quad z \to \infty \quad \text{or} \quad r \to \infty , \tag{3.2a}$$

$$c = 0 \qquad \text{for} \quad z = 0 \quad \text{and} \quad 0 < r < s , \tag{3.2b}$$

$$\frac{\partial c}{\partial z} = 0 \qquad \text{for} \quad z = 0 \quad \text{and} \quad s < r < \infty . \tag{3.2c}$$

The solution which obeys the first boundary condition is

$$c(r,z) = c(\infty) + \int_0^\infty A(\lambda) \, J_0 \, (\lambda r) \, \exp \, (-\lambda z) \, d\lambda , \tag{3.3}$$

where the J_v denote the Bessel functions of the first kind [1].

When the hitherto unknown function $A(\lambda)$ is chosen in such a way that the two other boundary conditions are satisfied one finds the dual integral equations

$$\int_0^\infty A(\lambda) \, J_0 \, (\lambda r) \, d\lambda = -c(\infty), \qquad (0 < r < s), \tag{3.4}$$

$$\int_0^\infty \lambda A(\lambda) \, J_0 \, (\lambda r) \, d\lambda = 0, \qquad (s < r < \infty). \tag{3.5}$$

This problem has been discussed in different contexts by various authors [2-4]. The solution is

$$A(\lambda) = - \frac{2 \, \sin \lambda \, s}{\pi \lambda} \, c(\infty), \tag{3.6}$$

which can be verified by substitution into (3.4,5) and using eqs. 11.4.38 and 11.4.35 of ref. 1 to evaluate the resulting integrals. The ligand current into the binding site is given by the integral

$$J = 2\pi D_T \int_0^s r \left[\frac{\partial c}{\partial z} \right]_{z=0} dr$$

$$= 4D_T c(\infty) \int_0^s r \, dr \int_0^\infty J_0(\lambda r) \, \sin \lambda s \, d\lambda$$

$$= 4D_T c(\infty)s , \tag{3.7}$$

where eq. 11.4.38 of [1] was used again. Hence in this case $\alpha = 4$. Combination of (3.3) and (3.6) shows that - just as in the previous model - the pertubation $c(r,z) - c(\infty)$ of the ligand concentration away from its asymptotic value at infinity is appreciable only in a region with a size of order s.

4. The electrostatic analog; the dumbbell-shaped binding site

If a binding site has a more complicated shape the calculation of the ligand current becomes a formidable problem which often cannot be solved rigorously. Yet one can invoke various approximations which will often lead to accurate results. In the next section we discuss the variational method which was developed by Goldstein, van Opheusden and the author [5,6]. First we discuss the electrostatic analog of the diffusion problem and apply it to a dumbbell-shaped binding site.

In order to demonstrate the formal (not physical!) connection with electrostatics we set

$$c = \left[1 - \frac{\phi}{\phi_0} \right] c(\infty) \tag{4.1}$$

where ϕ_0 is some constant. Substitution into (1.3-5) shows that $\phi(\vec{r})$ is a solution of

$$\Delta\phi = 0 \tag{4.2}$$

subject to the boundary conditions

$$\phi \to 0 , \qquad\qquad (r \to \infty) , \tag{4.3}$$

far from the binding site;

$$\phi = \phi_0 \tag{4.4}$$

on the binding site, and

$$\frac{\partial\phi}{\partial z} = 0 \tag{4.5}$$

everywhere on the plane of the membrane outside the binding site. The last boundary condition is automatically satisfied provided ϕ is defined on both sides of the membrane and the binding site below the membrane is defined as the mirror image of the binding site above the membrane. The equations (4.2-4) show that ϕ is the electrostatic potential outside a system of conductors with the same shape as the binding site, with $\phi = \phi_0$ on their surface.

The inward diffusive flux, J, into the binding site is given by the surface integral over the binding site

$$J = D_T \int \vec{\nabla}c \cdot d^2\vec{S} . \tag{4.6}$$

Because of the symmetry of the problem with respect to the plane of the membrane we can as well write

$$J = \frac{D_T}{2} \int \vec{\nabla}c \cdot d^2\vec{S} \tag{4.7}$$

where the surface integral extends over the binding site and its mirror image. Using (4.1) we can cast this in a form familiar from electrostatics

$$J = - \frac{Dc(\infty)}{2\phi_0} \int \vec{\nabla}\phi \cdot \vec{d^2s} \tag{4.8}$$

$$= - \frac{Dc(\infty)}{2\phi_0} \int \Delta\phi \cdot dV \tag{4.9}$$

where we used the theorem of Gauss and where the volume integral is extended over the interior of the binding site and its mirror image. Using Poisson's equation in the MKS system

$$\Delta\phi = -\rho/\varepsilon_0 , \tag{4.10}$$

where ρ is the charge density and ε_0 is the dielectric constant of the vacuum, the previous equation becomes

$$J = \frac{Dc(\infty)Q}{2\varepsilon_0\phi_0} \tag{4.11}$$

where Q equals the total charge enclosed by the binding sites when they are treated as conducting surfaces held at a constant potential ϕ_0. In terms of the capacitance C,

$$J = \frac{Dc(\infty)}{2\varepsilon_0} C . \tag{4.12}$$

Thus for receptors with a geometry for which the capacitance is known the last equation can be used to calculate the diffusive flux.

In order to demonstrate the power of the electrostatic analog we consider a dumbbell-shaped binding site, i.e. a binding site consisting of two identical hemispheres of radius s with centers separated by a distance d, where $d \geq 2s$. This problem was solved by Smythe [7] using the method of images; the essential steps are the following:

(a) The solution is written as the sum of two terms $\phi = \phi_1 + \phi_2$, both of which obey (4.2) and vanish at large distances from the binding site. Moreover $\phi_1 = \phi_0$ on the surface of sphere 1 and $\phi_1 = 0$ on the surface of sphere 2; for ϕ_2 the roles of the spheres are interchanged.

(b) In order to calculate ϕ_1 we note that the function ϕ_0 s/r, were r is the distance to the center of sphere 1, is a solution of Laplace's equation with the proper boundary condition on the surface of sphere 1, but not on the surface of sphere 2. In order to correct the boundary condition on the surface of sphere 2 we add a term which corresponds to a ligand source of the appropriate strength on the line connecting the two centers, at a distance s^2/d from the center of second sphere. This turns out to correct the boundary condition on sphere 2 but to spoil the boundary condition on sphere 1. This leads to another ligand sink to be placed on the line connecting the two centers, and so on.

(c) The contributions of the infinite series of alternating ligand sinks and sources of decreasing strengths can be summed and leads to the following expression for the flux into a dumbbell-shaped binding site

$$J = 4\pi D_T c(\infty) s \sum_{n=1}^{\infty} (-1)^{n+1} \frac{\sinh \beta}{\sinh n\beta} , \qquad (4.13)$$

$$\cosh \beta = \frac{d}{2s} . \qquad (4.14)$$

In the limit $d \to \infty$, in which the two half-spheres become independent, the flux approaches $4\pi D_T c(\infty) s$ which is twice the amount (2.5) for a single half-sphere. In the opposite limit, in which the spheres are made to touch, $d = 2s$ and the flux approaches the value

$$J = 4\pi D_T c(\infty) s \sum_{n=1}^{\infty} (-1)^{n+1} \frac{1}{n} = 4\pi D_T c(\infty) s \, \ell n \, 2 . \qquad (4.15)$$

Hence in this case α has the value $4\pi \, \ell n \, 2$.

As J is an increasing function of the separation d of the two half-spheres this calculation shows that clustering of the receptors in the cell membrane will decrease their ability to catch ligands.

5. The variational method for an arbitrary geometry: upper and lower bounds

Now consider the most general geometry: a cell of arbitrary shape with a membrane with any number of embedded receptors. We shall derive two variational principles for the total inward flux into the receptors

$$J = D_T \int_{S_0} \vec{\nabla} c \cdot d^2 \vec{S} , \qquad (5.1)$$

where S_0 denotes the whole surface; our derivation follows the one in ref. 6.

In order to keep the mathematics as simple as possible we enclose the cell in a second surface S_∞ at some large distance. Consider the collection of all sufficiently smooth functions $c_1(\vec{r})$ which have the properties:

$$c_1(\vec{r}) = c(\infty) \qquad \text{if } \vec{r} \in S_\infty , \qquad (5.2)$$

$$c_1(\vec{r}) = 0 \qquad \text{at the surface of the binding site,} \qquad (5.3)$$

$$\vec{\nabla} c_1(\vec{r}) \text{ is parallel to } S_0 \quad \text{at each point of } S_0 \text{ outside the binding sites.} \qquad (5.4)$$

For this class of functions we define the functional

$$J_1 [c_1] \equiv \frac{D_T}{c(\infty)} \int_V (\vec{\nabla} c_1)^2 \, d^3 V , \qquad (5.5)$$

where V denotes the volume enclosed between S_0 and S_∞.

Consider the function $c(\vec{r})$ for which J_1 is as small as possible. This function is a solution of the Euler-Lagrange equation $\Delta c = 0$ and as it obeys the boundary conditions (5.2-4) it is the solution of the diffusion problem for the ligands (provided we take the limit in which the surface S_∞ is moved to infinity in all directions). Hence the correct ligand distribution is found by minimizing the right hand side of (5.5).

Note that the numerical value of J_1 for $c_1 = c$ can be calculated as follows. Because

$$\text{div } c \, \vec{\nabla} \, c = (\vec{\nabla} c)^2 + c \Delta c = (\vec{\nabla} c)^2 \qquad (5.6)$$

one can write

$$J_1 [c] = \frac{D_T}{c(\infty)} \int_V \text{div } c\vec{\nabla}c \; d^3V = \frac{D_T}{c(\infty)} \int_{S_0+S_\infty} c\vec{\nabla}c \cdot d^2\vec{S}. \qquad (5.7)$$

On S_0 the product $c\vec{\nabla}c \cdot d^2S$ is always zero, either because of (5.3) or because of (5.4). As $c = c(\infty)$ on S_∞ one can write

$$J_1[c] = D_T \int_{S_\infty} \vec{\nabla}c \cdot d^2\vec{S} \; . \qquad (5.8)$$

But this also equals

$$J_1[c] = D_T \int_{S_0} \vec{\nabla}c \cdot d^2\vec{S} \qquad (5.9)$$

because $\Delta c = \text{div } \vec{\nabla}c = 0$ everywhere between S_0 and S_∞. Hence $J_1[c]$ simply equals the total ligand flux J.

Finally we should point out that J_1 is actually a minimum for $c_1 = c$, rather than just stationary. This follows by substitution of

$$c_1(\vec{r}) = c(\vec{r}) + \varepsilon(\vec{r}) \; , \qquad (5.10)$$

where ε takes small values. Eq. (5.5) takes the value

$$J_1[c_1] = J + \frac{D_T}{c(\infty)} \int (\vec{\nabla}\varepsilon)^2 \; d^3V \geq J \; . \qquad (5.11)$$

So, to summarize the results up till now, we found the variational principle

$$J = \min \frac{D_T}{c(\infty)} \int_V (\vec{\nabla}c_1)^2 \; d^3V \; , \qquad (5.12)$$

which provides upper bounds on the ligand flux into the receptors.

In order to derive a lower bound we note that eqs. (5.1) and (5.5) are both mathematically independent expressions for the ligand flux, given the concentration profile $c(\vec{r})$ and its gradient. We then have a whole class of expressions by considering linear combinations of these. One that will be particularly useful is

$$J_2[c_2] = \frac{D_T}{c(\infty)} \left\{ 2 \int_{S_0} c(\infty) \; \vec{\nabla}c_2 \cdot d^2\vec{S} - \int_V (\vec{\nabla}c_2)^2 \; d^3V \right\} \; . \qquad (5.13)$$

Again one considers variations ε around c_2, such that c_2 and $c_2 + \varepsilon$ both meet the correct boundary conditions. The variation of J_2 is found to be given by the expression

$$\delta J_2 = \frac{2D_T}{c(\infty)} \left\{ \int_{S_0} c(\infty) \, \vec{\nabla}\varepsilon \cdot d^2\vec{S} + \int_V \varepsilon \, \Delta c_2 \, d^3V \right\} - \frac{D_T}{c(\infty)} \int_V (\vec{\nabla}\varepsilon)^2 \, d^3V. \tag{5.14}$$

In order that J_2 be stationary one must now impose two conditions

$$\Delta c_2 = 0, \tag{5.15a}$$

$$\int_{S_0} \vec{\nabla}\varepsilon \cdot d^2\vec{S} = 0 . \tag{5.15b}$$

Thus, we must restrict ourselves to those variations of the distribution of the inward flux density over the receptor surface which are such that the total flux is fixed.

As the second variation is negative definite J_2 is maximal at its stationary point, so

$$J_2 \, [c_2] \leq J \, [c] \tag{5.16}$$

which provides lower bounds on the ligand flux. Combining this with (5.11) you get

$$J_2 \, [c_2] \leq J \, [c] \leq J_1 \, [c_1], \tag{5.17}$$

where the equality signs hold when c_1 and c_2 are equal to the exact solution c.

The complementary variational principles derived in this section were used by Goldstein, van Opheusden and the author to calculate upper and lower bounds for a variety of receptor geometries. For full details of these somewhat unwieldy calculations the reader might consult refs. 5 and 6. An application to the hemoglobin molecule has been reported by Beekwilder [8].

References to chapter III

[1] M. Abramowitz and I.A. Stegun. Handbook of Mathematical Functions (Dover, New York, 1972).
[2] J.D. Jackson. Classical Electrodynamics (Wiley, New York, 1963) § 3.12.
[3] I.N. Sneddon. Mixed Boundary Value Problems in Potential Theory (North-Holland, Amsterdam, 1966).
[4] T.L. Hill. Effect of rotation on the diffusion-controlled rate of ligand-protein association. Proc. Natl. Acad. Sci. USA 72 (1975) 4918-4922.
[5] B. Goldstein and F.W. Wiegel. The effect of receptor clustering on diffusion limited forward rate constants. Biophys. J. 43 (1983) 121-125.
[6] J.H.J. van Opheusden, F.W. Wiegel and B. Goldstein. Forward rate constants for receptor clusters: variational methods for upper and lower bounds. Biophys. Chem. 20 (1984) 237-248.
[7] W.R. Smythe. Static and Dynamic Electricity (McGraw-Hill, New York, 1968).
[8] J. Beekwilder. Toetsing van de toepasbaarheid van de variatiemethode op chemoreceptie: berekeningen aan de ligandenstroom naar hemoglobine. Unpublished D2 report, Department of Applied Physics, Twente University, 3 February 1984.

IV. THEORY OF ONE-STAGE CHEMORECEPTION

1. The method of the effective boundary condition

Once the ligand current into a single receptor is known, the next task is to develop a general theory for the rate of absorption of ligands by a cell of any shape that carries a large number of identical receptors in its cell membrane (cf. section I.4 (d)). In this chapter we address this problem, using the effective boundary condition method of DeLisi and Wiegel [1] and Wiegel [2], which can in principle be applied to cells of any shape, with an arbitrary distribution of receptors in the cell membrane. We shall include cases in which there are forces acting between the ligands and the cell and a flow field is present too.

Let $\vec{F}(\vec{r})$ denote the external force acting on a ligand at position $\vec{r}$ and let $\vec{v}(\vec{r})$ denote the velocity of the fluid flow field in $\vec{r}$. The ligand current density $\vec{J}(\vec{r},t)$ now consist of three terms: a diffusion term

$$- D_T \, \vec{\nabla} c ,$$

a drift term due to the effect of the external force

$$+ \frac{c}{f_T} \, \vec{F} ,$$

and a convective term

$$+ c\vec{v} .$$

Here f_T denotes the friction coefficient of a ligand, as discussed in chapter II. Hence

$$\vec{J} = - D_T \vec{\nabla} c + \frac{c}{f_T} \, \vec{F} + c\vec{v} , \tag{1.1}$$

and the concentration of the ligands must be solved from the partial differential equation

$$\frac{\partial c}{\partial t} = - \operatorname{div} \vec{J}$$

$$= D_T \Delta c - \frac{1}{f_T} \, (\vec{F} \cdot \vec{\nabla} c + c \operatorname{div} \vec{F}) - (\vec{v} \cdot \vec{\nabla} c + c \operatorname{div} \vec{v}) . \tag{1.2}$$

Usually the force is conservative, i.e. the force can be written as minus the gradient of some scalar potential ϕ

$$\vec{F} = - \vec{\nabla} \phi . \tag{1.3}$$

We shall always normalize ϕ in such a way that it equals zero at infinity

$$\phi(\infty) = 0 . \tag{1.4}$$

Also, in most cases the flow is incompressible, which can be expressed by

$$\operatorname{div} \vec{v} = 0 . \tag{1.5}$$

Using (1.3-5) eq. (1.2) can be written in a variety of ways. The equation has to be solved with the very complicated boundary conditions which express the fact that the binding sites are perfect absorbers of ligands and that the rest of the cell membrane is a perfect reflector.

The method of the effective boundary condition now relies on three order of magnitude estimates: (a) We notice that the size of the binding site is very small as compared to the radius of the cell

$$s \ll R , \tag{1.6}$$

cf. the estimates in section I.2. (b) The flux J_1 into a single receptor can be calculated from the ligand distribution in a vicinity (of linear dimension s) of the binding site by neglecting the external force. As the diffusion term in the current density (1.1) is of order $D_T c/s$ and the drift term of order Fc/f_T this will be true provided

$$Fs \ll D_T f_T = k_B T . \tag{1.7}$$

This means that the work which is performed by the external force when a ligand is moved over a distance equal to the radius of the binding site should be small as compared to the thermal energy of the ligand. (c) Similarly, we can calculate J_1 neglecting the convective effect of the flow. The convective term in (1.1) is of order cv, so this approximation is justified provided

$$sv \ll D_T . \tag{1.8}$$

Using $s \approx 5 \times 10^{-7}$ cm, $v \approx 15 \times 10^{-3}$ cm s^{-1} and $D_T \approx 10^{-6}$ cm^2 s^{-1} one finds $10^{-8} \ll 10^{6}$, so (1.8) is satisfied quite well.

The order of magnitude estimates (1.6-8) show that eq. (1.2) can be solved outside the cell, subject to the requirement that *at the cell's surface* the component of minus the ligand current density perpendicular to the membrane must be equal to $\alpha v D_T sc$, where v is the local density of binding sites (number of binding sites per unit area). This gives, in an obvious notation,

$$\{ D_T \vec{\nabla} c - \frac{c}{f_T} \vec{F} - c\vec{v} \}_\perp = \alpha v D_T sc . \tag{1.9}$$

Usually $\vec{v}$ is parallel to the cell membrane, so $\vec{v}_\perp = 0$ anyhow.

The method which uses the effective boundary condition (1.9) is essentially a form of asymptotic matching, in which the solution of the diffusion problem near to a binding site in the cell membrane is matched smoothly to the solution far away from the membrane. The reader might want to consult van Dyke [3] for the applications of this method in fluid mechanics.

2. The spherical cell

In order to demonstrate how the method of the effective boundary condition works we consider a spherical cell of radius R immersed in an unbounded medium. The cell carries N receptors in its outer membrane, which are uniformly distributed, so the number of binding sites per unit surface area is

$$v = \frac{N}{4\pi R^2} \cdot \tag{2.1}$$

The biological significance of a uniform receptor distribution was stressed by Purcell [4]: at the scale of a swimming microorganism the effect of the heat motion is so large that the cell cannot tell the difference between "up" and "down". Hence, if the cell is spherical it would be optimal to have its receptors distributed uniformly. We calculate the total number (J_N) of ligands assimilated by the cell, per unit of time, in a medium in which the ligand concentration approaches the constant value $c(\infty)$ at large distances from the cell. We shall first consider the stationary state, next the time dependent process of the relaxation of an initial ligand distribution to the stationary state. For convenience we ignore the effects of a flow field ($\vec{v}=0$) and we assume the force $\vec{F}$ to have spherical symmetry, i.e. the potential ϕ depends only on the distance to the center of the cell.

For this spherical case eq. (1.2) reads

$$\frac{\partial c}{\partial t} = D_T \left[\frac{\partial^2 c}{\partial r^2} + \frac{2}{r}\frac{\partial c}{\partial r} \right] + \frac{1}{f_T}\frac{d\phi}{dr}\frac{\partial c}{\partial r} + \frac{c}{f_T}\left(\frac{d^2\phi}{dr^2} + \frac{2}{r}\frac{d\phi}{dr} \right) . \tag{2.2}$$

In the stationary state $\partial c/\partial t = 0$, which equation can be written in the form (cf. refs. 1,2)

$$\frac{1}{r^2}\frac{d}{dr}\left[r^2 \frac{dc}{dr} + \frac{r^2 c}{k_B T}\frac{d\phi}{dr} \right] = 0 . \tag{2.3}$$

One integration gives

$$\frac{dc}{dr} + \frac{c}{k_B T}\frac{d\phi}{dr} = \frac{A}{r^2} \tag{2.4}$$

where A is a constant.

This equation simply expresses the fact that in the stationary state the ligand current should be the same through any spherical surface around the cell; this gives

$$\left[D_T \frac{dc}{dr} + \frac{c}{f_T}\frac{d\phi}{dr} \right] 4\pi r^2 = J_N \tag{2.5}$$

so the constant A is related to the total ligand current J_N by

$$A = \frac{J_N}{4\pi D_T} \cdot \tag{2.6}$$

The general solution of (2.4) which approaches $c(\infty)$ at large distances is found to have the form

$$c(r) = c(\infty) \exp \{- \phi(r)/k_B T\} -$$

$$- A \exp \{- \phi(r)/k_B T\} \int_r^\infty \frac{1}{\rho^2} \exp \{+ \phi(\rho)/k_B T\} d\rho . \tag{2.7}$$

Substitution of this equation for $r = R$ into the effective boundary condition (1.9), which now reads

$$D_T \frac{dc}{dR} + \frac{c(R)}{f_T} \frac{d\phi}{dR} = \alpha v \ D_T \ s \ c(R) \ , \tag{2.8}$$

gives the value

$$A = \frac{\alpha v \ s \ R^2 \ c(\infty) \ \exp \ \{- \ \phi(R)/k_B T\}}{1 + \alpha v s \ R^2 \ \{- \frac{\phi(R)}{k_B T}\} \ \int\limits_R^\infty \frac{1}{\rho^2} \ \exp \ \{+ \frac{\phi(\rho)}{k_B T}\} \ d\rho} \ . \tag{2.9}$$

The total ligand current into the whole cell follows upon substitution of the last equation and (2.1) into (2.6)

$$J_N = \frac{4\pi \ D_T \ \alpha s \ N \ c(\infty) \ \exp \ \{- \frac{\phi(R)}{k_B T}\}}{4\pi + \alpha s N \ \exp \ \{- \frac{\phi(R)}{k_B T}\} \ \int\limits_R^\infty \frac{1}{\rho^2} \ \exp \ \{+ \frac{\phi(\rho)}{k_B T}\} \ d\rho} \ . \tag{2.10}$$

This solves the problem set out at the beginning of this section. In the next section we consider two special cases and some of their biophysical implications.

3. Free diffusion and electrostatic attraction

For the case of free diffusion, which was considered by Berg and Purcell in their classic paper [I-34], the receptors have plane circular binding sites and no external force acts on the ligands. Substituting $\alpha=4$, $\phi=0$ into (2.10) the ligand current is found to be given by

$$J_N = 4\pi R D_T \ c(\infty) \ \frac{sN}{\pi R + sN} \ . \tag{3.1}$$

This formula was first derived by Berg and Purcell, using an altogether different method which has the drawback that it cannot be generalized to external forces, flow fields or other shapes of the cell.

The first factor $J_\infty = 4\pi R D_T \ c(\infty)$ is the ligand current into a perfectly absorbing sphere considered in chapter III. It is striking how fast this saturation value is reached when N increases. For example, J_N will equal 50% of the maximum current J_∞ if $N = \pi R/s$; using $R = 5 \times 10^4$ Å and $s = 50$ Å this gives $N \cong 3100$. For this value of N only a fraction

$$\frac{\pi s}{4R} \cong 0.8 \times 10^{-3} \tag{3.2}$$

of the area of the cell is occupied by binding sites. This implies that the cell can accomodate receptor systems for up to a hundred different types of ligands in less than 10% of its surface (each receptor system catching ligands at 50% of the largest possible rate) and still has more than 90% of the membrane surface available for activities other than chemoreception!

The remarkable efficiency of chemoreception is due to the erratic shape of the trajectories of a ligand: when the ligand hits the cell outside a binding site it will bounce back, but because of the chaotic nature of its motion it is likely to hit the membrane many times before it can escape from its vicinity, and one of those hits might hit a binding site. This is nowadays often called the fractal nature of the ligand trajectories [5], [I-4]. The fractal nature of the ligand trajectories is more obvious in a discrete approximation than in a continuous model like the one used in this monograph.

In the case of electrostatic attraction, first considered by DeLisi and Wiegel [1], the cell has a charge Q, the ligand a charge q of the opposite sign and

$$\phi(r) = \frac{qQ}{\varepsilon_0 r} , \tag{3.3}$$

where ε_0 is the dielectric constant of the extracellular medium. For plane circular binding sites of radius s eq. (2.10) gives a rate of ligand capture

$$J_N = 4\pi D_T c(\infty) \frac{sN\delta \ \exp \ (\delta/R)}{\pi\delta + s N \ \{\exp(\delta/R) -1\}} , \tag{3.4}$$

$$\delta = - \frac{qQ}{\varepsilon_0 k_B T} > 0 . \tag{3.5}$$

The dimensionless ratio δ/R is of the order of magnitude of the ratio between the energy needed to move a ligand from the cell surface to infinity, and the thermal energy. For $\delta/R \ll 1$ the ligand flux approaches the free diffusion value (3.1). If in the case $N_s = \pi R$ considered before the cell picks up a small amount of charge such that $\delta/R = 1$ the ligand current doubles from the value $2\pi R D_T \ c(\infty)$ to $4\pi R D_T \ c(\infty)$. Of course, this new value is still smaller than the saturation value of the flux in the presence of an electrostatic attraction. The latter quantity is given by

$$\lim_{N \to \infty} J_N = 4\pi D_T \ c(\infty) \ \delta \ \frac{\exp \ (\delta/R)}{\exp \ (\delta/R) \ - \ 1} \tag{3.6}$$

and hence in this case still larger than the saturation value in the absence of forces by a factor $\frac{e}{e \ - \ 1} \cong 1.6$.

4. Time dependent ligand currents

It should be clear from the previous three sections how the stationary state of the ligand current into a cell can be calculated. The method can be used for cells of any shape and forces and flows of any type. Often one also wants to know how some original ligand distribution relaxes into the stationary state in the course of time. This problem was recently considered by Geurts and Wiegel [6] whose treatment we follow in this section.

To be more specific we consider the case of free diffusion, i.e. we solve the time dependent equation (2.2)

$$\frac{\partial c}{\partial t} = D_T \left[\frac{\partial^2 c}{\partial r^2} + \frac{2}{r} \frac{\partial c}{\partial r} \right] . \tag{4.1}$$

Consider the case in which originally the ligand concentration has a constant value c_0 everywhere, i.e. the initial condition is

$$c(r,0) = c_0 \ , \ (R < r) . \tag{4.2}$$

The boundary condition at the cell surface is given at all times by (1.9), which now reads

$$\frac{\partial c}{\partial r} = \frac{Ns}{\pi R^2} c \quad , \quad (r = R, \, t > 0) \; .$$
(4.3)

If the function $c(r,t)$ is written in the form

$$c = c_0 - c_0 \; \frac{sN}{\pi R + sN} \; \frac{R}{r} \; (1-f)$$
(4.4)

one finds upon substitution into (4.1) that the unknown function $f(r,t)$ is the solution of

$$\frac{\partial f}{\partial t} = D_T \frac{\partial^2 f}{\partial r^2} \; ,$$
(4.5)

subject to the initial condition

$$f(r,0) = 1 \quad , \quad (R < r) \; ,$$
(4.6)

and to the boundary condition

$$\frac{\partial f}{\partial r} = \beta \, f \quad , \quad (r = R, \, t > 0) \; ,$$
(4.7)

$$\beta = \frac{\pi R + sN}{\pi R^2}$$
(4.8)

at the surface of the cell.

The advantage of working with the function f instead of c is that (4.5) has the form of the one-dimensional diffusion equation, for which many convenient methods of solution are known [7]. Application of these methods leads to the explicit solution

$$f(r,t) = \mathrm{erf} \left[\frac{r-R}{2\sqrt{D_T t}} \right] +$$

$$\left\{ 1 - \mathrm{erf} \left[\frac{r-R}{2\sqrt{D_T t}} + \beta \sqrt{D_T t} \right] \right\} \exp \left\{ \beta(r-R) + \beta^2 D_T t \right\} \, ,$$
(4.9)

where erf denotes the function

$$\mathrm{erf} \, z = \frac{2}{\sqrt{\pi}} \int_0^z e^{-t^2} \, dt \; .$$
(4.10)

It is straightforward, although somewhat tedious, to verify this solution by substituting it into the equations (4.5-7).

The time dependent ligand current is found to be given by

$$J_N(t) = 4\pi R^2 \, D_T \frac{\partial c}{\partial R} = 4\pi R D_T \, c_0 \frac{sN}{\pi R + sN} \; \cdot$$

$$\cdot \left[1 + \frac{sN}{\pi R} \left\{ 1 - \mathrm{erf}(\beta \sqrt{D_T t}) \right\} \exp \left(\beta^2 D_T t \right) \right] \; .$$
(4.11)

This shows how the stationary state (3.1) is approached: for $t \to \infty$ one can use the asymptotic formula

$$1 - \text{erf} (\beta \sqrt{D_T t}) \cong \frac{1}{\beta \sqrt{D_T t}} \exp (- \beta^2 Dt) \qquad (4.12)$$

to show that the large time behavior of the ligand capture rate is

$$J_N(t) \cong J_N(\infty) \left[1 + \frac{sN}{\pi R + sN} \frac{R}{\sqrt{\pi D_T t}} \right] , \quad (t \to \infty) . \qquad (4.13)$$

This shows a rather slow approach to the stationary value. In the opposite limit $t \to 0$ one finds

$$J_N(0) = J_N(\infty) (1 + \frac{sN}{\pi R}) = 4s \, ND_T c_0 , \qquad (4.14)$$

which is simply N times the capture rate of a single binding site. The full formula (4.11) describes the gradual transition form the initial stage in which the N receptors independently capture ligands, to the stationary state in which the receptors compete for the depleted ligand population surrounding the cell.

5. Ligand capture by saturating receptors

In this section we study the fictitious case of a cell involved in chemoreception; each time a receptor captures a ligand that receptor is blocked permanently. This situation is not common in chemoreception properly speaking but does occur in other applications of the formalism discussed here. For the spherical cell geometry without an external force the exact calculation of the number N(t) of unblocked receptors at time t is very difficult. This problem was analyzed by Geurts and Wiegel [8]. They showed that the ligand distribution outside the cell can be expressed in terms of an integral over the distribution at the surface of the cell. For the latter they derived a nonlinear integral equation which they solved numerically. In this way one can determine the time-dependent ligand current into the cell, and the average number of free receptors in the cell surface as a function of time.

The formalism in ref. [8] is quite complicated and for practical purposes one would like a simpler theory. Such a simplified approach is possible if one assumes that R^2/D_T is small as compared to the overall relaxation time. In this case one can use the following approximate equation

$$\frac{dN}{dt} = - 4\pi \, RD_T \, c(\infty) \frac{sN}{\pi R + sN} . \qquad (5.1)$$

The solution is

$$(N_0 - N) + \frac{\pi R}{s} \ell n \left[\frac{N_0}{N} \right] = 4\pi \, RD_T \, c(\infty)t , \qquad (5.2)$$

where N_0 denotes the number of unblocked receptors at $t = 0$ and ℓn the natural logarithm.

The cell becomes inert, i.e. unable to catch ligands, if N has dropped below some number of order unity. The last equation shows that the time needed for this to happen is

$$t_0 \cong \frac{\ell n \, N_0}{4s \, D_T c \, (\infty)} \, ,$$ (5.3)

which can of course be quite large when the concentration of ligands in the environment of the cell is small.

6. Comments on the case of a cylindrical cell

It was already remarked in sections I.2 (a) and I.3 (a) that many cells have a more or less cylindrical shape, so one would like to develop the theory of one stage chemoreception for an infinitely long circular cylinder. Here one should clearly distinguish the problems in the absence or presence of a flow field, as the mathematical treatment is quite different in the two cases, and somewhat tricky anyhow.

In the absence of a flow field the problem can be treated in a way similar to the treatment in the sections 1-5 of this chapter provided the ligand concentration is kept at the constant value c_0, not at infinity but at some large but finite distance R_1 from the axis of the cylinder. In cylindrical coordinates the case of free diffusion leads to the stationary state concentration profile

$$c(r) = c_0 \left\{ 1 - \frac{\alpha v s R \, \ell n \frac{R}{r}}{1 + \alpha v \, s R \, \ell n \frac{R_1}{R}} \right\} , \quad (R < r < R_1),$$ (6.1)

where R is the radius of the cylinder and $v = N/2\pi R$, with N the number of receptors per unit height. The total ligand flux per unit height equals

$$J_N = \frac{4 \, Ns \, c_0 \, D_T}{1 + \frac{4}{2\pi} \, Ns \, \ell n \frac{R_1}{R}} \, ,$$ (6.2)

where we used $\alpha = 4$.

The case in which a flow field is present is relevant to the detection of pheromones by the antenna receptors of moths like *Bombyx mori*. This problem has been studied in considerable detail by Murray [I-25] to whose monograph we refer for details.

7. The probabilities of capture and escape of a ligand

It was already mentioned in section I.4 (e) that various problems related to the capture (or escape) of a ligand by a single cell are somewhat related to the theory of one-stage chemoreception by that cell. For example, consider the model of a spherical cell used in sections 2-4 and a single ligand which at time t=0 is located a distance $r_0 > R$ from the center of the cell. One can now ask for the probability $P_c(r_0)$ that this ligand will eventually be captured by the cell, or for the probability $P_e(r_0) = 1 - P_c(r_0)$ that it will never be captured.

A fictitious experiment would consist of creating a stationary state in which the ligand concentration at $r = r_0$ is kept fixed at the value $c(r_0) = c_0$. Solving (2.4) with the two boundary conditions $c(r_0) = c_0$, $c(\infty) = 0$ one finds

$$c(r) = c_0 \frac{\exp\left\{-\frac{\phi(r)}{k_B T}\right\} \int_r^\infty \rho^{-2} \exp\left\{+\frac{\phi(\rho)}{k_B T}\right\} d\rho}{\exp\left\{-\frac{\phi(r_0)}{k_B T}\right\} \int_{r_0}^\infty \rho^{-2} \exp\left\{+\frac{\phi(\rho)}{k_B T}\right\} d\rho} , \qquad (r > r_0) . \tag{7.1}$$

The corresponding total outward ligand flux follows from (2.6)

$$J_{out}(r_0) = \frac{4\pi D_T\, c(r_0)}{\exp\left\{-\frac{\phi(r_0)}{k_B T}\right\} \int_{r_0}^\infty \rho^{-2} \exp\left\{+\frac{\phi(\rho)}{k_B T}\right\} d\rho} . \tag{7.2}$$

In the same way the concentration profile for $R < r < r_0$ follows from the solution of (2.4) under the two boundary conditions (2.8) and $c(r_0) = c_0$. From this concentration profile the total inward ligand flux $J_{in}(r_0)$ follows by means of (2.6). The resulting equations are somewhat messy; they simplify considerably in the limit $r_0 \downarrow R$, in which one studies the capture and escape of a ligand which is released just outside the surface of the cell.

In this case the outward flux follows from (7.2)

$$J_{out}(R) = \frac{4\pi D_T\, c(R)}{\exp\left\{-\frac{\phi(R)}{k_B T}\right\} \int_R^\infty \rho^{-2} \exp\left\{+\frac{\phi(\rho)}{k_B T}\right\} d\rho} . \tag{7.3}$$

The inward flux is given by $(4\pi R^2)$ times the value of the ligand current density at the surface of the cell. According to (1.9) or (2.8) the latter equals $\alpha \nu D_T s\, c(R)$, with $\nu = \dfrac{N}{4\pi R^2}$ one finds

$$J_{in}(R) = N\alpha D_T s\, c(R) . \tag{7.4}$$

Hence the probability that a ligand which is released at the surface of the cell will be captured by the cell is given by

$$P_c(R) = \frac{J_{in}(R)}{J_{in}(R) + J_{out}(R)} = \frac{N\alpha s\, \exp\left\{-\frac{\phi(R)}{k_B T}\right\} \int_R^\infty \rho^{-2} \exp\left\{+\frac{\phi(\rho)}{k_B T}\right\} d\rho}{4\pi + N\alpha s\, \exp\left\{-\frac{\phi(R)}{k_B T}\right\} \int_R^\infty \rho^{-2} \exp\left\{+\frac{\phi(\rho)}{k_B T}\right\} d\rho} . \tag{7.5}$$

In a similar way one finds for the probability that this ligand will escape forever

$$P_e(R) = \frac{J_{out}(R)}{J_{in}(R) + J_{out}(R)} = \frac{4\pi}{4\pi + N\alpha s \, \exp\left\{-\frac{\phi(R)}{k_B T}\right\} \int\limits_R^\infty \rho^{-2} \exp\left\{+\frac{\phi(\rho)}{k_B T}\right\} d\rho} \qquad .(7.6)$$

These expressions were first derived in [1]. Their relevance to the calculation of ligand-receptor rate constants has been discussed by DeLisi [9]. For free ligands (and plane circular binding sites) they simplify to

$$P_e(R) = \frac{4\pi R}{4\pi R + N\alpha s} = 1 - P_c(R) . \qquad (7.7)$$

For ligands which are subject to the electrostatic attraction (3.3) they become

$$P_e(R) = \frac{4\pi R}{4\pi R + N\alpha s \, \frac{R}{\delta} (e^{\delta/R} - 1)} = 1 - P_c(R), \qquad (7.8)$$

with δ defined by (3.5).

References to chapter IV

[1] C. DeLisi and F.W. Wiegel. Effect of nonspecific forces and finite receptor number on rate constants of ligand - cell bound receptor interactions. Proc. Natl. Acad. Sci. USA 78 (1981) 5569-5572.
[2] F.W. Wiegel. Diffusion and the physics of chemoreception. Phys. Reports 95 (1983) 283-319.
[3] M. van Dyke. Perturbation Methods in Fluid Mechanics (Parabolic Press, Stanford, 1975).
[4] E.M. Purcell. Life at low Reynolds numbers. Am. J. Phys. 45 (1977) 3-11.
[5] B.B. Mandelbrot. Fractals (Freeman, San Francisco, 1977).
[6] B.J. Geurts and F.W. Wiegel. Time-dependent ligand current into a single cell performing chemoreception. Biophys. Chem. 28 (1987) 7-12.
[7] H.S. Carslaw and J.C. Jaeger. Conduction of Heat in Solids (Clarendon Press, Oxford, 1959).
[8] B.J. Geurts and F.W. Wiegel. Time-dependent ligand current into a saturating cell performing chemoreception. Biophys. Chem. 31 (1988) 317-324.
[9] C. DeLisi. The biophysics of ligand-receptor interactions. Q. Rev. Biophys. 13 (1980) 201-230.

V. LIGAND CAPTURE BY A SYSTEM OF MANY CELLS

1. Coarse-grained description of a system of absorbing cells

In the present chapter we turn to problems which are related to a system of many cells, as well as to the time-dependence of ligand capture by such a system. The rough model calculations which follow are inspired by the fact that in the tissues of a living organism the cells which are involved in chemoreception will often not occur in isolation but in great numbers. This leads us to consider chemoreception by identical cells which are distributed in space with some number density m $(\vec{r},t)$ which can be a function of space and time. The treatment of this problem is particularly simple if the distance between cells is large as compared to the size of the cells, i.e. if

$$mR^3 \ll 1 \tag{1.1}$$

for spherical cells of radius R. In this case it is advantageous to define a coarse-grained ligand concentration

$$C(\vec{r},t) = \frac{1}{v} \int_V c(\vec{r}',t) \, d^3\vec{r}' \tag{1.2}$$

where the integration extends over a volume V which includes the point $\vec{r}$, and which is large enough to contain many cells, but small enough that $c(\vec{r}',t)$ is approximately constant inside V. The balance equation for the number of ligands gives (for the case in which flow fields and external forces are absent)

$$\frac{\partial C}{\partial t} = D_T \Delta C - 4\pi R \, D_T \beta \, m \, C. \tag{1.3}$$

The value of the constant β depends on the model used: $\beta = 1$ for a perfectly absorbing cell, $\beta = sN(\pi R + sN)^{-1}$ for the model of § IV.3 with free diffusion, $\beta = sN(\delta/R) \exp(\delta/R) [\pi\delta + sN \{\exp(\delta/R)-1\}]^{-1}$ for the case of electrostatic attraction studied there, and so on. The distribution of ligands throughout the tissue can be calculated by solving (1.3) under the appropriate initial- and boundary conditions.

A simple application is the stationary state of the ligand concentration throughout a tissue if ligands are replenished at the interface between the tissue and the rest of the organism. Putting the x-axis perpendicular to the plane interface and assuming $m = m_0 = $ constant throughout the tissue, the last equation simplifies to

$$\frac{d^2 C}{dx^2} = 4\pi R \beta m_0 C. \tag{1.4}$$

The solution

$$C(x) = C(0) \exp(-x \sqrt{4\pi R \beta m_0}), \tag{1.5}$$

which is independent of the value of the diffusion coefficient, shows that ligands penetrate the tissue over a distance of the order of magnitude $(4\pi R \beta m_0)^{-1/2}$. Of course, far more complicated geometries can be studied, but the basic physics will remain the same.

Another simple application is to the decay of a coarse-grained ligand distribution which is uniform at time $t = 0$. Eq. (1.3) now reads

$$\frac{dC}{dt} = - 4 \pi R D_T \beta m_0 C . \tag{1.6}$$

The solution

$$C(t) = C(0) \exp (-4 \pi R D_T \beta m_0 t) \tag{1.7}$$

implies an exponential decay on a time scale of the order of magnitude $(4 \pi R D_T \beta m_0)^1$. In section 3 of this chapter we shall consider this problem again and show that the simple exponential decay is just a rough approximation of the time dependence of the ligand distribution; more subtle effects will come to the fore. But first we study the question: when a ligand is originally placed at some position in the intercellular space, how much time lapses on the average till it is captured by one of the cells?

2. The mean time till ligand capture

Consider an arbitrary cell geometry, with or without attractive forces and a ligand that originally ($t = 0$) is located at position $\vec{r}_0$ outside the cells. Let $T(\vec{r}_0)$ denote the mean time that lapses till this ligand is captured by one of the cells. In this section we develop a general formalism to calculate the mean time till ligand capture.

First, one writes eq. IV.1.2 in the form

$$\frac{\partial c}{\partial t} = Lc; \quad L \equiv D_T \Delta - \frac{1}{f_T} \vec{F} \cdot \vec{\nabla} - \frac{1}{f_T} (\text{div } \vec{F}) - \vec{v} \cdot \vec{\nabla} - (\text{div } \vec{v}) . \tag{2.1}$$

The probability density $P(\vec{r},t|\vec{r}_0)$ to find the ligand near $\vec{r}$ at time t can be expanded in the orthonormalized eigenfunctions of the linear operator L

$$P(\vec{r},t|\vec{r}_0) = \sum_n \phi_n (\vec{r}) \phi_n^* (\vec{r}_0) \exp (-\lambda_n t) , \tag{2.2}$$

$$L\phi_n = -\lambda_n \phi_n . \tag{2.3}$$

The boundary conditions are that $\phi_n = 0$ on any binding site, and that $-D_T \vec{\nabla}\phi_n + \frac{1}{f_T} \vec{F} \phi_n + \vec{v} \phi_n$ will be parallel to the cell membranes everywhere outside the binding sites.

Second, one notes that the probability $W(t)$ that the ligand is not yet captured at time t is given by the integral

$$W(t) = \int_E P(\vec{r},t|\vec{r}_0)d^3\vec{r} \tag{2.4}$$

which extends over all the space (E) outside the cells. As the probability that the ligand will be captured during the time interval $(t, t+dt)$ is obviously given by $- \frac{\partial W}{\partial t} dt$, the mean time till capture equals

$$T(\vec{r}_0) = - \int_0^\infty t \frac{\partial W}{\partial t} dt = \int_0^\infty W(t) dt. \tag{2.5}$$

Substitution of (2.2) and (2.4) gives the eigenfunction expansion

$$T(\vec{r}_0) = \int_0^\infty dt \int_E d^3\vec{r} \sum_n \phi_n(\vec{r}) \phi_n^*(\vec{r}_0) \exp(-\lambda_n t)$$

$$= \sum_n \lambda_n^{-1} \phi_n^*(\vec{r}_0) \int_E \phi_n(\vec{r}) d^3\vec{r} . \tag{2.6}$$

In many cases of practical interest there is no flow field ($\vec{v} = \vec{0}$) and the external force on the ligands can be written as the derivative of a scalar potential

$$\vec{F}(\vec{r}) = - \vec{\nabla}\phi(\vec{r}) . \tag{IV.1.3}$$

It is easy to show that in this case all eigenvalues are real. Hence the previous equation gives

$$L\, T\,(\vec{r}) = - \int_E \sum_n \phi_n^*(\vec{r}) \phi_n(\vec{r}') d^3\vec{r}' = -1 . \tag{2.7}$$

This partial differential equation generalizes a result of ref. [I.34] to the case of external forces. The boundary conditions for T are the same as those for the eigenfunctions ϕ_n, as can be seen from eq. 2.6.

As an example of this formalism consider the mean time till capture for a single, perfectly absorbing spherical cell with freely diffusing ligands. In polar coordinates one should solve

$$\left[\frac{d^2}{dr^2} + \frac{2}{r} \frac{d}{dr} \right] T(r) = - \frac{1}{D_T} ; \tag{2.8}$$

under the boundary condition

$$T(R) = 0 \tag{2.9}$$

at the surface of the cell. In order to get a finite mean time till absorption one has to impose a reflecting spherical boundary condition at some distance $R_1 > R$, so

$$\frac{dT}{dr} = 0 , \qquad\qquad (r = R_1) . \tag{2.10}$$

The solution is

$$T(r) = \frac{1}{6D_T} (R^2 + \frac{2R_1^3}{R} - \frac{2R_1^3}{r} - r^2) . \tag{2.11}$$

There is of course an abundance of other geometries for which the mean time till the capture of a ligand can be calculated from eq. 2.7, either by an exact analytical solution or with some numerical procedure.

3. Examples of time-dependent problems

In the previous chapters we always studied the steady state of some situation which is relevant to chemoreception. For example, we studied the ligand flux into a cell, keeping the ligand concentration at large distances fixed; obviously time does not play a role in this problem. Yet, in many biophysical and biochemical experiments one observes the decay of a ligand population due to its capture by a system of traps. Some examples are the following.

A one-dimensional example would be the diffusion of a number of repressors along a single DNA molecule, followed by their binding to the corresponding operators. In this case one might be interested in the time-dependence of the number of bound repressor molecules.

A two-dimensional example is any experiment in which one observes the decay of a population of membrane proteins due to their capture by a system of traps. Usually the traps are in random, but fixed positions in the membrane, and each membane protein diffuses laterally in this membrane, till it hits a trap. An important case is the lateral diffusion of receptor proteins in the membrane of eukaryotic cells, and their capture by coated pits.

A three-dimensional example would be an experiment in which one follows how in an organism the population of antigens is depleted by their binding to macrophages. In the next section we discuss various ways to calculate the decay of the free (unbound) antigen population.

These experiments are usually interpreted under the assumption that the total number $N(t)$ of free ligands will decay as a "pure" exponential function of the form

$$N(t) \cong N_0 \exp\left[-\frac{t}{\tau_0}\right] , \qquad (3.1)$$

provided one considers the long-time behaviour of the decay. Here N_0 is a dimensionless constant (not necessarily equal to the original number $N(o)$ of free ligands) and τ_0 is a constant with the dimension of time. The pure exponential form (3.1) of the population decay is taken for granted by most authors, to such an extent that it almost has the status of a truism. This is probably due to the following "chemical" line of reasoning which immediately leads to (3.1): One argues that, if there are N free ligands at time t, and if there are fixed, absorbing traps with a spatial concentration

$$m = \frac{\text{number of traps}}{\text{volume of system}} = \frac{M}{V} , \qquad (3.2)$$

than the number of collisions between free ligands and traps, per unit of time, should be proportional to the product mN. Hence one would write down a kinetic equation of the form

$$\frac{dN}{dt} = -k_+ mN , \qquad (3.3)$$

which looks as little more than just the definition of the forward rate constant k_+. The solution of (3.3) has the form (3.1) with $N_0 = N(o)$ and

$$\tau_0 = (k_+ m)^{-1} . \qquad (3.4)$$

However, it is not at all obvious that one can always use a kinetic equation of the form (3.3). The *ad hoc* use of that equation implies that the extremely complicated "microscopic" diffusion of the ligands through the space in between the absorbing cells can always be described by nothing more than the "macroscopic" variable N. We shall analyze this question in more detail in the next section, where it is pointed out that (3.1) only holds when the traps are regularly spaced. We then analyze the case in which the traps are in fixed but random positions, and show that the long-time decay of the ligand distribution is of the fractional exponential form

$N(t) \cong N_0 \exp \{-(t/\tau)^{3/5}\}$ for a three dimensional system,
$\qquad N_0 \exp \{-(t/\tau)^{1/2}\}$ for a two dimensional system,
$\qquad N_0 \exp (-(t/\tau)^{1/3}\}$ for a one dimensional system.

We shall also briefly discuss the consequences of this point of view for the interpretation of the experiments.

4. Fractional exponential decay in the capture of ligands by randomly distributed traps

Consider a system which consists of M traps in a volume V. For convenience we take the traps to be perfectly absorbing spheres of radius a. The positions of the traps are fixed, and completely random, i.e. each trap can be placed anywhere in the volume with spatial probability density 1/V. At t = 0 there are N(o) ligands distributed uniformly throughout V. One asks for the long-time behavior of N(t). Following ref. [1] we consider this problem in three dimensions (the generalization of the solution to two- or one dimension is straightforward and discussed in [2,3]).

In order to grasp the physics of this diffusion process one should notice that there are two essential differences between these random traps and traps that are placed in regular positions: the former tend to cluster in patches in which their number density is somewhat higher than the average

$$m = \frac{M}{V} . \qquad (4.1)$$

Moreover, in between these patches one will find regions in which there are no traps at all. We shall call these regions "holes". So we shall visualize the system of random traps as a more-or-less uniform background with a density approximately given by (4.1), in which one finds, in various locations, holes of various shape and size.

The physics of the relaxation process is now the following. If the ligands have a diffusion coefficient D_T each one of them will diffuse over a distance of order $(D_T t)^{1/2}$ during time t. Those ligands which at t = 0 were situated in the regions of uniform trap density (call their number N_a) will be caught by the traps in a relatively short time. We shall show shortly that this part of the ligand population decays with a pure exponential of the form (3.1). However, those ligands which at t = 0 were situated in holes (N_b say) will survive much longer because, in order to be caught by a trap they first have to diffuse out of their hole, which will take a long time if the hole is large. We are going to show that this part of the ligand population decays with a fractional exponential $\exp -(t/\tau_b)^{3/5}$. So, putting everything together one finds that

$$N(t) \cong N_a \exp\{-t/\tau_a\} + N_b \exp\{-(t/\tau_b)^{3/5}\}, \quad (t \gg \tau_b). \tag{4.2}$$

As $N_b \ll N_a$ but $\tau_b \gg \tau_a$ the relaxation process is dominated by the first term for relatively short times ($\tau_a \ll t \lesssim \tau_a \log \frac{N_a}{N_b}$), but it is dominated by the second term for long times ($t \gg \tau_b$). In other words: the experimentalist should see a relaxation process that starts as a pure exponential but gradually transforms itself into a fractional exponential.

Before embarking upon the details of the calculation one should note that the fractional exponential behavior of the form $\exp\{-a\,(t/\tau)^b\}$, but with various values of the constants a and $0 < b < 1$, is found experimentally in a great variety of complex systems. These include mechanical relaxation, dielectric relaxation, ionic conductivity relaxation, spin-lattice relaxation, luminescence relaxation, and various relaxation processes in electronic hopping, magnetic systems and entangled polymer systems. For an overview of both the experimental and theoretical work in this field the reader is referred to the proceedings of a recent conference [4]. At the time of writing there is no consensus why the fractional exponential form of relaxation is so universal that it appears in physical systems of the most diverse nature. Rajagopal and the author [5] have speculated that it simply reflects a universal property of the heat bath, but this explanation is far from satisfactory. Our present model of ligand capture by randomly distributed traps has the advantage that the physical origin of this "anomalous" behavior can be shown quite clearly and that the theory can be developed analytically in considerable detail. We now turn to the calculation of the distribution of the hole size.

The holes can have a variety of shape and size. According to the principles of statistical physics the probability to find a hole with volume v should be proportional to the Boltzmann factor $\exp(-\frac{E}{k_B T})$, where k_B again denotes Boltzmann's constant, T the absolute temperature and E the amount of work needed to create the hole. Thermodynamics tells you that this energy equals $E = pv$ where $p = \frac{M}{V} k_B T$ equals the "pressure" in an ideal gas of M particles (traps) in a volume V. Collecting these results one finds that the probability to find a hole of volume v is proportional to

$$(\text{probability}) = (\text{constant}) \exp\left[-\frac{M}{V} v\right]. \tag{4.3}$$

An alternative way (essentially a Poisson distribution argument) to derive this is to note that the positions of the traps are statistically independent. Hence the probability that the first trap is located outside the volume v equals $1 - \frac{v}{V} \cong \exp(-\frac{v}{V})$ and the probability that this holds for all M traps is the Mth power of this expression, which leads to (4.3).

For calculational convenience we shall assume that all holes are spherical. Hence, for the total number $H(s)ds$ of holes with a radius between s and $s + ds$ we shall use the expression

$$H(s) = H_0 \frac{4\pi M}{V} s^2 \exp\left[-\frac{4\pi M}{3V} s^3\right]. \tag{4.4}$$

Here H_0, which denotes the total number of holes in the system, will be proportional to the total volume of the system. The specific value of H_0 depends on the precise definition of a hole and on the lower cutoff in the size of a hole. We do not know how to calculate H_0 a priori, so it will stay in the equations as the only adjustable parameter of the present theory.

In order to study the decay of those ligands which at $t = 0$ are located inside a hole we consider a spherical hole of radius s, surrounded by a more-or-less uniform distribution of traps at density m. For $t = 0$ the ligand concentration is a constant c_0 inside the hole and vanishes outside the hole. For $t > 0$ the ligands diffuse outside the hole and are annihilated by the traps. One has to calculate the decay of this ligand population asymptotically for $t \to \infty$. (Note that these ligands are only part of the total initial uniform ligand population in the system, namely those which at $t = 0$ are located inside this particular hole!)

Let the ligand distribution for $t > 0$ be denoted by $c(r,t)$ and use spherical coordinates around the center of the hole. The diffusion of the ligands can be described by

$$\frac{\partial c}{\partial t} = D_T \, \Delta \, c \, , \qquad\qquad (0 < r < s) \, , \qquad\qquad (4.5a)$$

$$\frac{\partial c}{\partial t} = D_T \, \Delta \, c - 4 \, \pi \, a \, D_T \, m \, c \, , \qquad (r > s) \, . \qquad\qquad (4.5b)$$

Here $a = \beta R$ in the notation of eq. (1.3) and Δ denotes the Laplace operator. The general solution will have the form of an eigenfunction expansion. If the spectrum has at least one discrete state (i.e. if the hole is large enough for the ground state to be a bound state) the long-time behaviour of the solution is

$$c(r,t) \cong d_0 \varphi_0(r) \exp(-\lambda_0 t) \, , \qquad (t \gg \frac{1}{\lambda_0}) \, , \qquad\qquad (4.6)$$

where d_0 is a constant, φ_0 denotes the ground state and $\lambda_0(s)$ the corresponding eigenvalue. In this case the ligand population $N(s,t)$ under consideration will decay like

$$N(s,t) \cong N_0(s) \exp\{-\lambda_0(s)t\} \, , \qquad (t \gg \frac{1}{\lambda_0}) \, , \qquad\qquad (4.7)$$

where

$$N_0(s) \cong 4\pi \, d_0 \int_0^\infty \varphi_0(r) \, r^2 \, dr \, . \qquad\qquad (4.8)$$

We proceed to calculate the ground state eigenvalue λ_0, which sets the scale for this relaxation process.

As the ground state will be spherically symmetric it can be solved from

$$D_T \left[\frac{d^2}{dr^2} + \frac{2}{r} \frac{d}{dr} \right] \varphi_0 + \lambda_0 \varphi_0 = 0 \, , \qquad (0 < r < s) \, , \qquad\qquad (4.9a)$$

$$D_T \left[\frac{d^2}{dr^2} + \frac{2}{r} \frac{d}{dr} \right] \varphi_0 - (4\pi \, a \, m \, D_T - \lambda_0) \, \varphi_0 = 0 \, , \quad (r > s) \, . \qquad\qquad (4.9b)$$

Substitution of

$$\varphi_0(r) = \frac{\psi(r)}{r} \tag{4.10}$$

gives

$$\frac{d^2\psi}{dr^2} + \frac{\lambda_0}{D_T} \psi = 0 , \qquad (0 < r < s) , \tag{4.11a}$$

$$\frac{d^2\psi}{dr^2} - (4\pi \, a \, m - \frac{\lambda_0}{D_T}) \, \psi = 0 , \qquad (r > s) . \tag{4.11b}$$

There are boundary conditions at $r = 0$, at $r = s$ and at $r = \infty$. The boundary condition at $r = 0$ requires $\frac{\psi}{r}$ to be finite, hence

$$\psi(r) = A \, \sin \sqrt{\frac{\lambda_0}{D_T}} \, r , \qquad (0 < r < s) . \tag{4.12a}$$

The boundary condition at $r = \infty$ requires $\frac{\psi}{r} \to 0$ for $r \to \infty$. Hence

$$\psi(r) = B \, \exp \, (- \sqrt{4\pi \, a \, m - \frac{\lambda_0}{D_T}} \, r) , \qquad (r > s) . \tag{4.12b}$$

The values of the two constants A and B follow from the boundary condition at $r = s$, where φ_0 and $\frac{d\varphi_0}{dr}$ must be continuous. Hence ψ and $\frac{d\psi}{dr}$ must be continuous at $r = s$. This gives the set of equations

$$A \, \sin \sqrt{\frac{\lambda_0}{D_T}} \, s = B \, \exp \, (- \sqrt{4\pi \, a \, m - \frac{\lambda_0}{D_T}} \, s) , \tag{4.13a}$$

$$A \sqrt{\frac{\lambda_0}{D_T}} \cos \sqrt{\frac{\lambda_0}{D_T}} \, s = -B \sqrt{4\pi \, a \, m - \frac{\lambda_0}{D_T}} \, \exp \, (- \sqrt{4\pi \, a \, m - \frac{\lambda_0}{D_T}} \, s). \tag{4.13b}$$

Taking the ratio and calling

$$\xi \equiv \sqrt{\frac{\lambda_0}{D_T}} \, s \tag{4.14}$$

one finds the condition

$$\xi \, \cotg \, \xi = -\sqrt{4\pi \, a \, m \, s^2 - \xi^2} , \tag{4.15}$$

from which the spectrum can be solved. The properties of the eigenvalues follow in a straightforward way if one plots both sides of the last equation as functions of ξ. The right hand side is of course part of a circle of radius $\sqrt{4\pi \, a \, m \, s^2}$. One finds in this way that there is a solution (i.e. there is a bound state) if

$$\sqrt{4\pi \, a \, m \, s^2} > \frac{\pi}{2} ; \tag{4.16}$$

there are two bound states if $\sqrt{4\pi \, a \, m \, s^2} > \frac{3}{2} \pi$; and there will generally be n bound states if

$$\sqrt{4\pi \, a \, m \, s^2} > (n + \frac{1}{2}) \, \pi . \tag{4.17}$$

One also finds that the lowest bound state has a ξ value very near to π, so $\xi \cong \pi$ provided ams^2

is large as compared to $\pi/16$. Combination with (4.14) gives

$$\lambda_0(s) \cong \frac{\pi^2 D_T}{s^2}, \qquad\qquad (ams^2 >> \tfrac{\pi}{16}). \qquad\qquad (4.18)$$

It would not be hard to give a better approximation for $\lambda_0(s)$ for $\tfrac{\pi}{16} \leq ams^2$, but this is not needed for what follows. It would also be straightforward, although somewhat tedious, to calculate the constant $N_0(s)$ from (4.8), but this too is not needed. All one needs is the asymptotic form of the decay of this ligand population

$$N(s,t) \cong \tfrac{4}{3} \pi s^3 c_0 \exp\left[-\frac{\pi^2 D_T t}{s^2} \right], \qquad\qquad (4.19)$$

provided the hole is large enough to have at least one bound state. We shall now use this result to study the decay of those ligands which initially are located inside the large holes.

Now consider all those ligands which at $t = 0$ were situated in holes with radii

$$s > s_0 \equiv \sqrt{\frac{\pi}{16\,a\,m}}, \qquad\qquad (4.20)$$

that is: in holes large enough to have a bound state. This population consists of

$$N_h(t) = \int_{s_0}^{\infty} N(s,t)\, H(s)\, ds \qquad\qquad (4.21)$$

ligands. Combination of (4.4) and (4.13) gives

$$N_h(t) \cong \tfrac{1}{3} (4\pi)^2 c_0 m H_0 \int_{s_0}^{\infty} s^5 \exp\left[-\frac{4\pi}{3} ms^3 - \pi^2 \frac{D_T t}{s^2} \right] ds, \qquad\qquad (4.22)$$

which we shall show to have the fractional exponential form of the second term on the right-hand side of eq. (4.2).

The evaluation of the integral is an elementary exercise in the application of Laplace's method. If one introduces the new variable of integration

$$x \equiv t^{-1/5} s \qquad\qquad (4.23)$$

the last equation becomes

$$N_h(t) \cong \tfrac{16}{3} \pi^2 c_0 m H_0 t^{6/5} \int_{s_0 t^{-1/5}}^{\infty} x^5 \exp\{-t^{3/5} f(x)\}\, dx, \qquad\qquad (4.24)$$

where

$$f(x) = \frac{4\pi}{3} m x^3 + \pi^2 D_T x^{-2}. \qquad\qquad (4.25)$$

Obviously this function has a minimum where

$$\frac{df}{dx} = 4 \pi m x^2 - 2 \pi^2 D_T x^{-3} = 0. \qquad\qquad (4.26)$$

The solution is

$$x_0 = \left[\frac{\pi D_T}{2m} \right]^{1/5} . \tag{4.27}$$

The second derivative at this point is

$$\frac{d^2 f}{dx^2} = 8 \pi m x_0 + 6 \pi^2 D_T x_0^{-4} = 20 \pi m \left[\frac{\pi D_T}{2m} \right]^{1/5} , \tag{4.28}$$

which is positive. Hence for $t \to \infty$ one can write

$$N_h(t) \cong \frac{16}{3} \pi^2 c_0 m H_0 t^{6/5} x_0^5 \int_0^\infty \exp \{-t^{3/5} f(x_0) - \frac{1}{2} t^{3/5} f''(x_0) (x-x_0)^2\} dx$$

$$\cong \frac{16}{3} \pi^2 c_0 m H_0 t^{6/5} x_0^5 \exp \{-t^{3/5} f(x_0)\} (2\pi)^{1/2} t^{-3/10} \{f''(x_0)\}^{-1/2} ,$$

$$(t \to \infty) . \tag{4.29}$$

As

$$f(x_0) = \frac{10}{3} \pi m \left[\frac{\pi D_T}{2m} \right]^{3/5} \tag{4.30}$$

combination of the last four equations gives the long-time decay law

$$N_h(t) \cong \alpha' c_0 H_0 m^{-2/5} D_T^{9/10} t^{9/10} \exp (-\beta' m^{2/5} D_T^{3/5} t^{3/5}) , \tag{4.31}$$

where α' and β' are the somewhat unlikely looking numerical constants

$$\alpha' = \frac{8}{3} 2^{-2/5} 5^{-1/2} \pi^{+29/30} , \tag{4.32}$$

$$\beta' = \frac{10}{3} 2^{-3/5} \pi^{+8/5} . \tag{4.33}$$

Of course, the factor $t^{9/10}$ is meaningless as compared to the factor $\exp(-t^{3/5})$, so (4.31) has the form of a fractional exponential of the type studied by various authors (for a review of the theoretical work cf. [6]). In the remaining part of this section we need only analyze: (1) the decay of the population of ligands which for $t=0$ are located in "small" holes; (2) the decay of those ligands located near traps in the regions of more or less uniform trap density. We shall show that both populations decay as a pure exponential.

For holes radii larger than the order of magnitude $m^{-1/3}$ of the average distance between traps, but smaller than the s_0 of eq. 4.20, there are no bound states, i.e. the equations 4.9a,b have no solutions which satisfy the boundary conditions at $r = 0$, $r = s$ and $r = \infty$. In this case the ligands will diffuse away from their hole and at time t the concentration profile $c(r,t)$ should have a spatial scale of order $(D_T t)^{1/2}$. A glance at 4.5b shows that the term $D_T \Delta c$ is now negligeable as compared to the term $4\pi a D_T mc$. Hence, for t larger than some interval t_0 equation 4.5b can be replaced by

$$\frac{\partial c}{\partial t} \cong - 4\pi a D_T m c , \qquad (r > s, t > t_0) , \tag{4.34}$$

which has the solution

$$c(r,t) = c(r,t_0) \exp \{-4 \pi a D_T m (t-t_0)\} \ . \tag{4.35}$$

Consequently the population $N_{sh}(t)$ of the ligands which originally were located in these small holes will, for long times, decay as a pure exponential function

$$N_{sh}(t) \cong (constant) \exp (-4 \pi a D_T m t), \qquad (t > t_0) \ . \tag{4.36}$$

Hence this ligand population only contributes to the first term on the right-hand side of eq. 4.2.

Finally we consider the population of ligands which at $t = 0$ were located outside the holes, i.e. in the areas where the trap density is more or less uniform. The elementary unit of space to be modelled is now a single trap, surrounded by a fixed volume which we shall take to be a sphere of a fixed radius R such that

$$\frac{4}{3} \pi R^3 = \frac{V}{M} = m^{-1} \ . \tag{4.37}$$

As in this case only the region $a < r < R$ matters we can still study the relaxation of the ligands in this spherical region, due to capture by the central trap, using eqs. 4.5, 6, 9a, 10, 11a. The solution of the eigenvalue problem is

$$\psi(r) = A \sin \sqrt{\frac{\lambda_0}{D_T}} r + B \cos \sqrt{\frac{\lambda_0}{D_T}} r \ , \qquad (a < r < R) \ . \tag{4.38}$$

In this case there are two boundary conditions: First, the concentration should vanish at $r = a$ due to the trap being a perfect spherical absorber of ligands; this gives

$$A \sin \sqrt{\frac{\lambda_0}{D_T}} a + B \cos \sqrt{\frac{\lambda_0}{D_T}} a = 0 \ . \tag{4.39}$$

Second, $\varphi'(r)$ should vanish at $r = R$, where one can imagine a reflecting boundary condition. This gives the condition

$$R \psi'(R) = \psi(R) \tag{4.40}$$

or

$$A \sin \sqrt{\frac{\lambda_0}{D_T}} R + B\cos \sqrt{\frac{\lambda_0}{D_T}} R = \sqrt{\frac{\lambda_0}{D_T}} R \left[A\cos \sqrt{\frac{\lambda_0}{D_T}} R - B\sin \sqrt{\frac{\lambda_0}{D_T}} R \right] \ . \tag{4.41}$$

Calling

$$\sqrt{\frac{\lambda_0}{D_T}} a \equiv p \ , \ \sqrt{\frac{\lambda_0}{D_T}} R \equiv q \tag{4.42}$$

one finds a non-trivial solution if and only if

$$\begin{vmatrix} \sin p & \cos p \\ \sin q - q \cos q & \cos q + q \sin q \end{vmatrix} = 0 \ . \tag{4.43}$$

Evaluation of the determinant and use of the addition theorem for the trigonometric functions gives the condition

$$tg\ (q-p) = q \ , \tag{4.44}$$

from which the eigenvalues, and especially the ground state can be solved.

By drawing the curves of tg(q-p) and $q = (q-p) + p$ as functions of q - p the reader easily convinces himself that the eigenvalue spectrum consists of bound states only. For small values of p the ground state will be close to $(q-p) = 0$, so one can use the power series expansion of the tangent

$$tg\ x = x + \frac{1}{3}\ x^3 + \frac{2}{15}\ x^5 + \ ... \ . \tag{4.45}$$

Taking the first two terms only one finds

$$\lambda_0 = \frac{3\ a\ D_T}{(R-a)^3} \ . \tag{4.46}$$

As a will be small as compared to R one can simplify this further; combination with (4.37) gives

$$\lambda_0 \cong \frac{3\ a\ D_T}{R^3} = 4\ \pi\ a\ D_T\ m \ . \tag{4.47}$$

This, of course, implies that this whole ligand population will, for long times, decay with a pure exponent

$$N_{tr}(t) \cong (\text{constant})\ \exp\ (-4\ \pi\ a\ D_T\ m\ t) \ . \tag{4.48}$$

The decay rate of this subpopulation of ligands is actually equal to the decay rate (4.36) of the ligand population in small holes, at least to leading order. There are small correction terms in the exponents of (4.36) and (4.48) which are not quite identical, but these corrections are at present experimentally unobservable anyhow.

In this section we have demonstrated a ligand decay of the form (4.2), where the pure exponential comes from the ligands which originally were near traps or inside small holes, and where the fractional exponential comes from the ligands which were originally situated inside the large holes.

It is not hard to verify that the fractional exponential has the form $N_2\ \exp\ \{-\ (t/\tau_2)^{1/2}\}$ for a two-dimensional system (cf. ref. 2) and $N_1\ \exp\{-\ (t/\tau_1)^{1/3}\}$ for a one-dimensional system (cf. ref. 3), where N_1, N_2, τ_1, τ_2 have the appropriate values.

From the derivations of our results it should be clear that one expects the fractional exponential decay law to appear for all those systems in which the positions of the traps are sufficiently random to allow the occurrence of holes large enough to have a bound state. If the positions of the traps are weakly random, i.e. if the holes which occur are too small to have bound states, the decay will be a pure exponential.

Before we close this section it should be pointed out that ideas similar to those discussed here have been used by Ovchinnikov and Zeldovich [7] in the study of bimolecular reaction kinetics, as well as by a variety of authors in other contexts. Some of these papers have been referenced in [1-3].

References to chapter V

[1] F.W. Wiegel. Fractional exponential decay in the capture of ligands by randomly distributed traps. Physica 139A (1986) 209-222

[2] F.W. Wiegel en J.H.J. van Opheusden. Fractional exponential decay of a membrane population due to capture by coated pits. Biophys. Chem. 28 (1987) 1-5

[3] B.J. Geurts and F.W. Wiegel. Fractional exponential decay in the capture of ligands by randomly distributed traps in one dimension. Bull. Math. Biol. 49 (1987) 487-494

[4] K.L. Ngai and G.B. Wright. Relaxations in complex systems (Office of Naval Research, Arlington, Virginia, 1985)

[5] A.K. Rajagopal and F.W. Wiegel. Nonexponential decay in relaxation phenomena and the spectral characteristics of the heat bath. Physica 127A (1984) 218-227

[6] A.K. Rajagopal and K.L. Ngai. Models of temporal stretched exponential relaxation in condensed matter systems. Ref. 4 pg. 275-301

[7] A.A. Ovchinnikov and Y.B. Zeldovich. Role of density fluctuations in bimolecular reaction kinetics. Chem. Phys. 28 (1978) 215-218.

VI. DIFFUSION AND FLOW IN THE CELL

1. Membrane diffusion coefficients

In chapters II-V we developed the theory of one-stage chemoreception, in which a ligand can only be absorbed by a cell by a direct hit on the binding site of the receptor molecule. In chapter VIII the theory will be extended to incorporate two-stage capture processes in which the ligand is first incorporated in the cell membrane and then diffuses laterally in the plane of the membrane till it hits a binding site. Actually, two-stage chemoreception is only one of a variety of processes which occur at the surface of the living cell and in which the lateral translational - or rotational diffusion of proteins plays an essential role. It is for this reason that the experimental determination of the relevant diffusion coefficients has been pursued vigorously during the last decade [37-44]. Experimental values of the the lateral translational diffusion coefficient $(D_T{}')$ range from 10^{-8} to 10^{-11} cm^2 s^{-1}. For the rotational diffusion coefficient $(D_R{}')$ of proteins embedded in the cell membrane one measures values in the range from 10^5 to 10^3 s^{-1}.

The physiological time scale set by membrane diffusion can be illustrated by the following numerical examples. The square of the circumference of a spherical cell is typically of order $(2\pi R)^2 \approx 10^{11}$ Å^2 using Table I.1. Substituting this number into the left hand side of

$$<\vec{r}^2> = 4D_T{}'t \tag{1.1}$$

one finds that a protein with a diffusion coefficient $D_T{}' \approx 10^{-8}$ cm^2 s^{-1} will diffuse once around the cell in about four minutes.

In this section we shall outline the way in which the lateral diffusion coefficients $(D_T{}', D_R{}')$ of a ligand immersed in the cell membrane can be calculated from "first principles", which in this case means hydrodynamics. This problem will be studied using the model of section I.2(c) in which a membrane protein is represented by a cylindrical disk of thickness h and radius a which is constrained to move in the plane of the membrane. The lipid bilayer fraction of the membrane is represented by a layer of continuous fluid of thickness h and viscosity η. The membrane is embedded in a fluid of viscosity η'. For a hard disk this problem was studied by Saffman and Delbrück [9,10]. For permeable polymer coils or porous comlexes of cross-linked proteins it was studied in a series of papers by Wiegel and Mijnlieff which are reviewed in a monograph [II.5]. The asymptotic analysis by Saffman of the translational lateral diffusion coefficient of a hard disk will be outlined shortly. For the record only we note that the rotational lateral diffusion coefficient is much easier to calculate; in the lowest order of approximation one finds

$$D_R{}' = \frac{k_B T}{4\pi\eta h a^2} . \tag{1.2}$$

With the typical values h $\approx$ 4 x 10^{-7} cm, a $\approx$ 2 x 10^{-7} cm, $\eta \approx$ 2 g cm^{-1} s^{-1}, $k_B T \approx$ 4 x 10^{-14} cm^2 g s^{-2} one finds $D_R{}' \approx 10^5$ s^{-1}, in fair agreement with the experiments.

In order to sketch Saffman's asymptotic analysis for $D_T{}'$ one uses Cartesian coordinate (x,y,z) with the z-axis along the axis of the cylinder and the x,y plane parallel to the membrane surface. The membrane is located at $-h < z < 0$ and the intra- and extracellular fluid at $z < -h$ and $z > 0$.

First, the pressure p and velocity $\vec{v} = (v_1, v_2, v_3)$ of the fluid at $z > 0$ and $z < -h$ have to be solved from

$$-\vec{\nabla}p + \eta'\Delta\vec{v} = 0 , \qquad \mathrm{div}\ \vec{v} = 0, \tag{1.3a,b}$$

under the boundary conditions that at large distances from the z-axis $v_1 \to -v_0$, $v_2 \to 0$, $v_3 \to 0$.

Second, the pressure P and velocity $\hat{V}$ of the membrane ($-h < z < 0$) are functions of x and y only, as the membrane flow will be strickltly two-dimensional to a very good approximation. They have to be solved from

$$-\vec{\nabla}P + \eta\Delta\hat{V} + \frac{2\eta'}{h} \left(\frac{\partial\vec{v}}{\partial z}\right)_{z=0} = 0, \qquad \mathrm{div}\ \hat{V} = 0. \tag{1.4a,b}$$

The third term represents the force of viscous friction exerted by the intra- and extracellular fluid on the membrane. The boundary conditions are that for large values of x or y the velocity approaches $V_1 = -v_0$, $V_2 = 0$. The continuity of the flow fields inside and outside the membrane are expressed by the condition

$$\hat{V}(x,y) = \vec{v}(x,y,0) . \tag{1.5}$$

For a hard disk one also needs a boundary condition at the surface of the disk, which takes the form

$$\hat{V}(x,y) = 0 \quad \text{if} \quad x^2 + y^2 = a^2 . \tag{1.6}$$

The asymptotic analysis makes use of a singular perturbation technique (c.f. ref. II.4) which works only provided the parameter

$$\theta = \frac{h\eta}{a\eta'}, \tag{1.7}$$

is very large as compared to unity. As full details can be found in refs. 10 and II-5 we only outline the basic idea. For $r \gg a$ the hard wall boundary condition (1.6) can be replaced by adding a sharply peaked force density $\vec{F}$ to the left hand side of 1.4a, with the x- and y-components

$$F_1 = \frac{F}{\pi h r} \delta(r) , \qquad F_2 = 0 . \tag{1.8a,b}$$

Here F denotes the magnitude of the total force which the protein exerts on the membrane fluid. The resulting set of equations, with the appropriate boundary conditions at infinity, can be solved analytically. The solution is called the outer asymptotic expansion of the flow field.

For $r \ll h\eta/\eta'$ the third term in the left hand side of (1.4a) can be neglected with respect to the second term. The solution of the resulting equations, with the appropriate boundary conditions along the z-axis, is called the inner asymptotic expansion.

In the case in which $\theta \gg 1$ both asymptotic expansions hold for $a \ll r \ll h\eta/\eta'$. This enabled Saffman to determine the value of the unknown constant F. In this way one finds for the translational lateral diffusion coefficient

$\theta = \dfrac{\eta h}{\eta' a}$	NUM	SAF
5/3	2.7	-30.1
3	1.9	3.8
7	1.2	1.5
15	0.86	0.94
29	0.68	0.72
61	0.55	0.57
125	0.46	0.47

Table VI.1

Values of $k_B T (2\pi \eta h D_T')^{-1}$ for various values of θ (left column), as calculated numerically (middle column) or from Saffman's asymptotic formula (1.9) (right column). The parameter $\sigma = \infty$; this corresponds to a hard disk. The numerical accuracy is expected to be about one unit in the last decimal place. Data are taken from ref. [15].

$$D_T' \cong \frac{k_B T}{4\pi\eta h} (-\gamma + \ell n\theta) , \qquad (\theta \gg 1) , \qquad (1.9)$$

where $\gamma = 0.5772$ denoted Euler's constant.

Saffman's work has been generalized by various authors. In a remarkable paper Hughes, Pailthorpe and White [11] calculate further terms in the asymptotic expansion (also c.f. Hughes [12]). They find

$$D_T' = \frac{k_B T}{4\pi\eta h} \left[-\gamma + \ell n\theta + \frac{8}{\pi\theta} - \frac{2}{\theta^2} \ell n\theta + 0(\theta^2) \right].$$ (1.10)

Actually, these authors can in principle calculate the full result through the following steps: (a) The boundary value problem defined by (1.3-6) is reduced to a set of dual integral equations. (b) These are transformed into a single integral equation using Erdélyi-Kober operators (c.f. Sneddon, reference [III.3]). (c) The integral equation is transformed into an equation for an infinite matrix. (d) This matrix equation is solved numerically.

In the context of chemoreception one also needs D_T' and D_R' for more intricate geometries. For example, in many cases of biological interest proteins in the cell membrane form aggregates as a result of some cross-linking process. For example, immunoglobulin molecules in the lymphocyte membrane can be cross-linked by multivalent antigens outside the membrane. In this way a patch consisting of hundreds or thousands of such molecules can form. Such an aggregate can diffuse laterally as a single entity in the membrane, and one should calculate the appropriate diffusion coefficient.

In order to do so one can again describe the aggregate as a cylindrical disk of radius a. When the disk moves laterally in the membrane the lipids can flow through the space in between the "stems" of the immunoglobulin molecules.

Hence one should give the disk a certain constant hydrodynamic permeability k_0, c.f. the discussion of the hydrodynamic permeability in section II.1. Writing

$$\sigma \equiv \frac{a}{\sqrt{k_0}} \qquad\qquad (1.11)$$

one finds for the lateral diffusion coefficients

$$D_T' \cong \frac{k_B T}{4\pi\eta h} \left\{ -\gamma + \ell n\, \theta + \frac{2}{\sigma^2} + \frac{I_0(\sigma)}{\sigma I_1(\sigma)} \right\}, \; (\theta \gg 1), \qquad\qquad (1.12)$$

$$D_R' \cong \frac{k_B T}{4\pi\eta h a^2} \frac{I_0(\sigma)}{I_2(\sigma)}, \qquad\qquad (\theta \gg 1), \qquad\qquad (1.13)$$

where the I_n denote the modified Bessel functions, which are tabulated in [III-1]. The derivations of these asymptotic formulae have been given in the monograph II-5; the original references are [13,14].

A problem with all the asymptotic results quoted in this subsection is that it is not clear how fast the asymptotic behavior is reached, i.e. how good are they for the typical values $\theta = 100$, $\sigma = 1$? In order to answer this question unambiguously Heringa, Wiegel and van Beckum [15] solved the linearized hydrodynamic equations numerically for a wide range of the relevant parameters θ and σ. For the special case $\sigma = \infty$, which corresponds to Saffman's model with an impermeable disk, the numerical results for the dimensionless quantity $k_B T(2\pi\eta h D_T')^{-1}$ are listed in Table VI.1. A glance at the table shows that Saffman's formula is already fairly accurate for θ as small as 15. Note that for the special case $\sigma = \infty$ the numerical results of refs. [11] and [15] should be identical; at present no such comparison has been completed yet.

2. Theory versus experiments on membrane diffusion

In this section we very briefly compare the theory with the experiments on membrane diffusion. If one substitutes into the asymptotic formulae (1.9, 10) the same typical values for the parameters as were used in (1.2), one finds the order of magnitude estimate $D_T' \approx 2 \times 10^{-8}$ cm^2 s^{-1}. However, experimental values [1-8] for D_T' range from 10^{-8} to 10^{-11} cm^2 s^{-1}. What is wrong? Possible deficiencies of Saffman's model have been discussed by a variety of authours [16, 17-19]; the main ones are the following.

(a) The simplest approximation of membrane diffusion is to describe it as a stricktly two-dimensional diffusion process. However, as was pointed out in this context by Buas [17], macroscopic hydrodynamic calculations on the surface of a sphere are plagued by theoretical difficulties, which lead to ambiguities in the definition of the transport coefficients. Of course, in Saffman's model the two-dimensional membrane is coupled to the three-dimensional intra- and extracellular fluid, but because of the smallness of the coupling constant $\theta^{-1} \approx 10^{-2}$ this coupling is weak. This weak coupling in turn causes the disturbance of the flow field around a protein to extend beyond the positions of other nearby proteins. As a result, for actual experiments, the movements of different proteins in the same cell membrane are not independent. To the author's knowledge this effect has not been analyzed theoretically.

(b) Bloom [20] has suggested that certain proteins in membranes have a "fluid-like" outer region which provides an approximate match with the lipid membrane. This effect could be taken into account by altering the boundary condition in Saffman's model. Zero tangential stress leads to a term $+ \frac{1}{2}$ added inside the bracket of (1.9) [10], and hence gives a larger diffusion coefficient than predicted by (1.9). As the experimental values of D_T' are smaller than the values predicted by (1.9) it is unlikely that Bloom's suggestion would improve the situation in this respect.

(c) If the protein binds to and dissociates from the cytoskeleton or other submembraneous binding sites the ensuing diffusion process will be slowed down considerably. If we can describe this binding by a single dissociation constant K, the effective lateral translational diffusion coefficient was estimated by Elson and Reidler [21] to be given by

$$D_T' = D_F' \frac{KS}{N+KS} + D_S' \frac{N}{N+KS} , \tag{2.1}$$

where S is the surface area of the cell, N the average number of free binding sites, D_F' the translational lateral diffusion coefficient of free proteins and D_S' the translational lateral diffusion coefficient of proteins bound to submembraneous structures. At the time of writing there is increasing evidence that tethering does play a substantial role in membrane diffusion (c.f. [19]).

(d) Another possibility is suggested by Owicki and McConnell [22]. The membrane may not be in the pure fluid phase, but in a mixed state in which regions characterized by a high density and a very small diffusion coefficient D_S' are immersed in a fluid phase with much higher diffusion coefficient D_F'. The observed Brownian motion of a protein actually consists of an alternation of rapid and slow diffusion in the two types of environment. The effective diffusion coefficient is shifted down towards D_S' and even anisotropy can arise [23]. The effective lateral diffusion coefficients given in [22] for a model where the membrane consists of layers with alternating slow and fast diffusion are

$$D_{//} = fD_F' + (1 - f)D_S' , \tag{2.2}$$

$$\frac{1}{D_\perp} = \frac{f}{D_F'} + \frac{1-f}{D_S'} , \tag{2.3}$$

respectively for the effective diffusion parallel and perpendicular to the layers, where f is the surface fraction of fluid membrane.

(e) More realistic than the layered structure considered in [22] is a model in which the lipid fraction of the membrane is in a state in which two of its phases coexist (c.f. the discussion in subsection I-2(b)). On a "mesoscopic" scale (finer than a macroscopic scale but coarser than the molecular scale) the membrane will consist of regions which are in one or the other pure phase. This leads to the statistically isotropic membrane model, which consists of regions (with slow and fast diffusion) of arbitrary shape and size such that on a scale compared to the size of the regions the properties are isotropic. This model, which was investigated by Wiegel and Heringa [18], is related to the problem of the effective conductivity of polycrystalline materials. One finds [24,25,18] that the effective lateral diffusion coefficient D', if the surface fraction of fluid membrane equals f, obeys the functional equation

$$D'(f,D_F',D_S')D'(1-f,D_F',D_S') = D_F'D_S' . \tag{2.4}$$

This relation is not sufficient to calculate the effective lateral diffusion coefficient, unless $f = 1/2$, in which case one finds

$$D'(1/2,D_F',D_S') = \sqrt{D_F'D_S'} . \tag{2.5}$$

Hence, if D_S'/D_F' is of order 10^{-4} the effective diffusion coefficient is smaller than the diffusion coefficient $D_F' \approx 10^{-8}$ cm^2 s^{-1} in the fluid phase by a factor $\sqrt{D_S'/D_F'}$ of order 10^{-2}; this gives $D' \approx 10^{-10}$ cm^2 s^{-1}, in the experimental range.

3. Flow in the cell membrane: cap formation on lymphocytes

The outer membrane of the cell is not a passive entity; even in a state in which the cell as a whole is at rest the lipids and membrane proteins are being recycled continuously. It was first noticed by Bretcher that this process could induce lateral flow patterns in the cell membrane (for a review see [26]). As the flow is essentially generated by the removal of "old" molecules and the insertion of "new" ones, the resulting flow pattern is completely determined, in the stationary state, by the geometry of the cell and of the sites of removal and insertion, and by the rate of turnover. In sections 3 and 4 we shall develop the theory for two specific cases which are probably extremes of what happens in actual cells: (a) The cell membrane is a sphere; old lipids are removed at only one specific site and new lipids are inserted at random positions throughtout the whole cell surface. (b) The cell has the shape of a pancake, i.e. the upper half of the cell membrane has the shape of a circle; old lipids are removed at random positions throughout the membrane and new lipids are inserted uniformly along the circumference of the cell. The theory for case (a) was developed by Wiegel [27] and for case (b) by Goldstein, Wofsy and Echavarria-Heras [28] and by Goldstein and Wiegel [29]. The present section is devoted to case (a) and the next section to case (b).

Consider a spherical cell of radius R (c.f. section I.2(a)1). It is convenient to use spherical coordinates θ,φ on its surface in such a way that the specific point where old lipids are removed through endocytosis corresponds to the "North Pole" $\theta = 0$. New lipids are inserted at random positions on the membrane in such a way that, in the stationary state, a fraction α of the total area is renewed per unit of time. Hence α is a rough measure for the intensity of the lipid metabolism of the cell. As a result of these two processes one finds a local "Bretscher" flow with a velocity $v(\theta)$ which is directed tangentially to the membrane, in the direction of decreasing values of θ. As the lipid bilayer flows as an incompressible fluid one finds

$$v(\theta) = \alpha R (1 + \cos\theta)/\sin \theta. \tag{3.1}$$

The average value of v over the cell surface is

$$<v> = (4\pi R^2)^{-1} \int_0^{\pi} v(\theta)\ 2\pi R^2\ \sin\theta\ d\theta = \frac{\pi}{2}\ \alpha R\ . \tag{3.2}$$

Bretscher gives $<v> \cong 5 \times 10^{-6}$ cm s^{-1} as a typical average velocity.

It is now straightforward to calculate the potential energy Φ of a membrane protein at position θ. Following ref. [27] and [II-5] one finds

$$\Phi(\theta) = f_T' \int_0^{\theta} \alpha R^2\ \frac{1 + \cos\theta'}{\sin\theta'}\ d\theta'$$

$$= 2\alpha R^2 f_T'\ \ell n\ (\sin \frac{\theta}{2}) + \text{constant}\ , \tag{3.3}$$

where f_T' denotes the translational friction coefficient of sections 1 and 2 of this chapter.

Hence, according to the principles of statistical physics the number density $\rho(\theta)$ of the diffusing membrane proteins (number per unit area) is given by

$$\rho(\theta) = \rho(\pi)\ (\sin \frac{\theta}{2})^{-2\alpha R^2/D_T'}\ , \tag{3.4}$$

where $\rho(\pi)$ denotes their density at the "South Pole" and where the Einstein relation (II.1.2) was used to express f_T' in terms of D_T'.

The last equation can be used as a rough approximation to the exact distribution of membrane proteins on the cell membrane of - for example - a lymphocyte. This density has the remarkable property that its integral over the whole membrane surface will diverge if $2\alpha R^2/D_T' \geq 2$. This divergence implies that a membrane protein on such a lymphocyte, if picked at random, will be found in an infinitesimal vicinity of $\theta = 0$ with probability 1. The resulting clustering phenomenon can be interpreted to mean that the membrane proteins form a "cap" at $\theta = 0$. In this way one has derived a rough quantitative criterion for cap formation.

$$(\text{cap formation}) \longleftrightarrow (\alpha R^2 \geq D_T')\ . \tag{3.5}$$

From a biophysical point of view this criterion implies that the cell can force its membrane proteins to cap either by increasing its lipid metabolism (larger α), or by decreasing their laterial diffusion coefficient (which itself results from an increase in membrane viscosity η, c.f. eq. 1.9).

Finally we note that the effects of the excluded volume of the membrane proteins can be taken into account with the methods of section II.-3; c.f. ref. [30]. If each membrane protein effectively blocks an area a^2 one finds that (3.4) must be replaced by

$$\rho(\theta) = a^{-2} \left\{ 1 + e^{-\mu}\ (\sin \frac{\theta}{2})^{2\alpha R^2/D_T'} \right\}^{-1}\ , \tag{3.6}$$

wher $e^{-\mu}$ is a parameter which has to be chosen in such a way that the total number of proteins equals N, so

$$2\pi R^2 \int_0^{\pi} \rho(\theta)\ \sin\theta\ d\theta = N\ . \tag{3.7}$$

Cap formation now shows up in the following way. At the North Pole the protein concentration equals $\rho(\theta) = a^{-2}$, hence the proteins are always close packed in that vicinity. With increasing θ their concentration decreases monotonously to a minimum of $a^{-2} (1 + e^{-\mu})^{-1}$ at the South Pole. For $2\alpha R^2 > D_T'$ the value of the protein concentration stays very near to the close packed value in a wide region around $\theta = 0$; for $2\alpha R^2 < D_T'$ this is not the case and $\rho(\theta)$ shows a peaked cusp at $\theta = 0$. Hence as one can identify the first case with the presence of a cap and the second case with the absence of a cap one has the criterion.

$$\text{(cap formation)} \longleftrightarrow (\alpha R^2 > \tfrac{1}{2} D_T') \ . \tag{3.8}$$

Note that (3.8) differs by a factor 1/2 from the previous criterion (3.5): the excluded volume effect makes it easier for cap formation to occur.

4. Flow in the cell membrane: cell surface protein distribution on spreading cells

When certain cells (for example giant HeLa cells) are deposited on a glass plate they tend to spread themselves out, taking the form of a more or less circular, rather flat pancake. Bretscher has suggested that on such "spreading" cells the insertion of new cell membrane components (lipids or proteins) occurs at the periphery of the cell, that is: uniformly along the circumference of the circle. Both receptors and lipids will be carried by diffusion and convection to small circular structures called coated pits, where they aggregate and next are internalized. These coated pits occur more or less uniformly over the entire surface of the cell.

It should be clear that this recycling process is equivalent to a flow pattern in the lipid component of the cell membrane; the flow originates at the circumference and its velocity is directed radially inwards. The proteins in the membrane, which are originally inserted at the circumference, are swept towards the center of the cell by the flow (convection). Moreover, the usual process of membrane diffusion, discussed in sections 1 and 2, is active, so the actual distribution of the proteins is the outcome of the competition between convection and diffusion. The resulting protein distribution is non-uniform. Experimentally such non-uniform distributions have been observed for the receptor proteins for the following ligands: low density lipoprotein, ferritin, transferrin, asialoglycoproteins, α-2-macroglobulin; c.f. ref. [29] for references to the original papers.

The coated pits into which the lipids and proteins aggregate are small circular invaginations of the surface, which become deeper in the course of time and are eventually internalized by the cell. They are approximately randomly distributed over the surface. Thus, endocytosis occurs uniformly over the cell surface, but exocytosis occurs only at the periphery.

It should be pointed out that not all membrane proteins aggregate into coated pits, some of them are excluded from coated pits, e.g. the θ and H63 antigens on mouse fibroblast cells [29]. Hence the quantitative theory to be developed shortly should enable one to predict the distribution of both types of proteins. In this section we follow the work reported in [29].

Consider a thin, spread cell, and model its surface as a two-dimensional disc of radius R.

Membrane lipids and surface proteins are inserted at the circumference of the disc. Coated pits that internalize lipids and internalize or exclude surface proteins, are uniformly distributed over the area of the disc.

Let $v(r)$ denote the magnitude of the velocity of the lipid flow (directed towards the origin!), at a distance r from the center of the disc. Consider a circle of radius r on the surface of the cell. The lipid area within this circle is πr^2, so if a fraction α_m of the lipids are internalized per unit of time the velocity must be such that

$$2\pi r \ v(r) = \alpha_m \pi r^2 . \tag{4.1}$$

This gives for the velocity of the lipid flow field

$$v(r) = \frac{\alpha_m}{2} r . \tag{4.2}$$

Note that it follows from the definition of α_m that a single lipid has a probability $\alpha_m dt$ to be internalized during the infinitesimal time interval dt. Hence the probability that this specific lipid will "live" till t and be internalized during (t, t + dt) equals

$$p(t) \ dt = \exp(-\alpha_m t) \ \alpha_m dt . \tag{4.3}$$

The last equation implies that the mean time which a specific lipid spends on the cell surface before being internalized by a coated pit is given by

$$\tau_m = \int_0^\infty t \ p(t) \ dt = \frac{1}{\alpha_m} , \tag{4.4}$$

so (4.2) can also be written as

$$v(r) = \frac{1}{2\tau_m} r . \tag{4.5}$$

This flow field is directed towards the center. Note that there are no singularities in the velocity, in contrast to the case of the previous section where the velocity tends to ∞ at the North Pole of the lymphocyte, c.f. eq. (3.1).

From the flow field one can immediately derive the distribution of those cell surface proteins that are excluded from coated pits, i.e. which are not recycled by the cell. These particles are driven to the center of the cell by the flow, while diffusion tends to disperse them, as in the case discussed in the previous section. The energy of such a protein at position r is

$$E(r) = f_T' \int_0^r v(r') \ dr' = \frac{f_T'}{4\tau_m} r^2 \tag{4.6}$$

where again f_T' is the frictional coefficient for lateral movement. In the steady state the particles assume the Boltzmann distribution for thermal equilibrium, hence the protein concentration (number per unit of area) is given by

$$c(r) = c(0) \exp(- \frac{r^2}{4D_T'\tau_m}) , \tag{4.7}$$

where the Einstein relation was used once more and where D_T' denotes the membrane diffusion coefficient as discussed in the first two sections of this chapter. Hence the theory predicts that for proteins which are excluded from coated pits the concentration will be a Gaussian, being maximal at the cell center and decreasing towards the periphery of the spreading cell. If on giant HeLa cells one could find a protein with such a distribution the experiment would strongly support Bretcher's proposal that there is an inward membrane flow.

Now consider the case of cell surface proteins that recycle through capture by a coated pit. Apart from at the periphery of the cell, where they are inserted, their concentration $c(r,t)$ is the solution of

$$\frac{\partial c}{\partial t} = -\text{div }\vec{j} - \alpha_p\, c \tag{4.8}$$

where $\vec{j}$ is the protein current density and α_p the fraction of the proteins internalized per unit of time. As

$$\vec{j} = -D_T'\, \vec{\nabla}c + c\vec{v}\ , \tag{4.9}$$

$$\alpha_p = \frac{1}{\tau_p}\ , \tag{4.10}$$

with τ_p the average life time of a protein in the cell membrane, one finds

$$\frac{\partial c}{\partial t} = D_T'\,\Delta c - \vec{v}\cdot\vec{\nabla}c - c\,\text{div }\vec{v} - \frac{1}{\tau_p}\,c\ . \tag{4.11}$$

Because of the circular symmetry of the problem the solution will depend on r only. Transformation to polar coordinates and substitution of (4.5) gives

$$\frac{\partial c}{\partial t} = D_T'\left[\frac{\partial^2 c}{\partial r^2} + \frac{1}{r}\frac{\partial c}{\partial r}\right] + \frac{r}{2\tau_m}\frac{\partial c}{\partial r} - \left(\frac{1}{\tau_p} - \frac{1}{\tau_m}\right)c. \tag{4.12}$$

Here we used $\text{div }\vec{v} = v/r + dv/dr$ for radially symmetric flow fields.

It is more convenient to use as the independent variables the dimensionless quantities

$$x = \frac{r}{\sqrt{2D_T'\tau_m}}\ , \quad \tau = \frac{t}{2\tau_m}\ , \tag{4.13}$$

in terms of which the differential equation becomes

$$\frac{\partial c}{\partial \tau} = \frac{\partial^2 c}{\partial x^2} + \left(x + \frac{1}{x}\right)\frac{\partial c}{\partial x} - \gamma c\ , \tag{4.14}$$

where

$$\gamma \equiv 2\left(\frac{\tau_m}{\tau_p} - 1\right)\ . \tag{4.15}$$

In the stationary state the left hand side of (4.14) is zero. The solution is

$$c(x) = c(0)\left\{1 + \frac{\gamma}{2^2}\,x^2 + \frac{\gamma(\gamma-2)}{2^2\,4^2}\,x^4 + \frac{\gamma(\gamma-2)(\gamma-4)}{2^2\,4^2\,6^2}\,x^6 + ...\right\} \tag{4.16}$$

as can easily be verified by substitution.

It is perhaps instructive to consider the solution in the limits in which convection c.q.

diffusion dominates. The case of pure convection is the limit $D_T' \rightarrow 0$. In this case the transformation (4.13) is not defined, so it is easier to go back to the original equation (4.12) which in this case reads

$$\frac{r}{2\tau_m} \frac{dc}{dr} = \left[\frac{1}{\tau_p} - \frac{1}{\tau_m}\right] c \qquad (4.17)$$

in the stationary state. The solution is

$$c(r) = c(R) \left(\frac{r}{R}\right)^\gamma , \qquad\qquad (D_T' = 0) , \qquad\qquad (4.18)$$

where $c(R)$ is the protein density at the periphery. From the definition (4.15) of γ it is seen that $c(r)$ increases from center to periphery if $\tau_m > \tau_p$, i.e. if proteins are recycled faster than lipids. If proteins are recycled slower than lipids $c(r)$ decreases towards the periphery from a weak singularity at the origin. In this case the integral

$$2\pi \int_0^R r\, c(r)\, dr = \frac{2\pi R^2 c(R)}{\gamma + 2} \qquad (4.19)$$

is always finite, because $\gamma + 2 = 2\tau_m/\tau_p > 0$, so no cap formation can occur in this flow field, in contrast with the case discussed in the previous section.

In the opposite case, in which diffusion dominates and lipid flow is negligeable, one has to take the limit $\tau_m \rightarrow \infty$ in (4.12). The stationary state has to be solved from

$$\frac{\partial^2 c}{\partial r^2} + \frac{1}{r} \frac{\partial c}{\partial r} = \frac{c}{D_T' \tau_p} . \qquad (4.20)$$

The solution which is finite in the origin is

$$c(r) = c(0) \, I_0 \left[\frac{r}{\sqrt{D_T' \tau_p}} \right] , \qquad (4.21)$$

where I_0 denotes the modified Bessel function [III-1]. This function increases monotonically from $r = 0$ to $r = R$.

In the general case in which both convection and diffusion are significant the full series (4.16) has to be taken into account numerically. The value of the constant $c(0)$ is determined by the outer boundary condition. If S_0 denotes the number of new proteins inserted into the upper half of the spreading cell at the boundary, per unit of time and per unit of length, then from (4.9) we find the requirement

$$+ D_T' \frac{\partial c}{\partial r} + \frac{r}{2\tau_m} c = S_0 \qquad (r = R) . \qquad (4.22)$$

In terms of the dimensionless variable x of (4.13) this reads

$$\frac{\partial c}{\partial x} + xc = S_0 \sqrt{\frac{2\tau_m}{D_T}} , \qquad \left[x = \frac{R}{\sqrt{2 D_T' \tau_m}} \right] , \qquad (4.23)$$

which shows that for a cell of a given size, for which $R/\sqrt{2D_T'\tau_m}$ has a fixed value, the value of $c(0)$ will be proportional to $S_0 \sqrt{2\tau_m/D_T'}$. Full numerical results and a comparison with the experimental data can be found in [29].

References to chapter VI

[1] R.J. Cherry. Rotational and lateral diffusion of membrane proteins. Biochim. Biophys. Acta 559 (1979) 289-327.
[2] M. Shinitzky and P. Henkart. Fluidity of cell membranes - current concepts and trends. Int. Rev. Cytol. 60 (1979) 121-147.
[3] M.M. Poo, J.W. Lam, N. Orida and A.W. Chao. Electrophoresis and diffusion in the plane of the cell membrane. Biophys. J. 26 (1979) 1-22.
[4] D.E. Golan and W. Veatch. Lateral mobility of band 3 proteins in the human erythrocyte membrane studied by fluorescence photobleaching recovery. Proc. Natl. Acad. Sci. USA 77 (1980) 2537-2541.
[5] B.A. Smith, W.R. Clark and H.M. McConnell. Anisotropic molecular motion on cell surfaces. Proc. Natl. Acad. Sci. USA 76 (1979) 5641-5644.
[6] M. Edidin, T. Wei and S. Holmberg. The role of membrane potential in determining rates of lateral diffusion in the plasma membrane of mammalian cells. Ann. N.Y. Acad. Sci. 339 (1980) 1-7.
[7] M.P. Scheetz, M. Schindler and D.E. Koppel. Lateral mobility of integral membrane proteins is increased in spherocytic erythrocytes. Nature 285 (1980) 510-512.
[8] W.L.C. Vaz, K. Jacobson, E.S. Wu and Z. Derzko. Lateral mobility of an amphipathic apolipoprotein, Apo-C-111, bound to phosphatidylcholine bilayers with and without cholesterol. Proc. Natl. Acad. Sci. USA 76 (1979) 5645-5649.
[9] P.G. Saffman and M. Delbrück. Brownian motion in biological membranes. Proc. Natl. Acad. Sci. USA 73 (1975) 3111-3113.
[10] P.G. Saffman. Brownian motion in thin sheets of viscous fluid. J. Fluid Mech. 73 (1976) 593-602.
[11] B.D. Hughes, B.A. Pailthorpe and L.R. White. The translational and rotational drag on a cylinder moving in a membrane. J. Fluid Mech. 110 (1981) 349-372.
[12] B.D. Hughes. Ph.D. Thesis, Australian National University, 1980, unpublished.
[13] F.W. Wiegel. Rotational friction coefficient of a permeable cylinder in a viscous fluid. Phys. Lett. 70A (1979) 112-113.
[14] F.W. Wiegel. Translational friction coefficient of a permeable cylinder in a sheet of viscous fluid. J. Phys. A12 (1979) 2385-2392.
[15] J.R. Heringa, F.W. Wiegel and F.P.H. van Beckum. Friction coefficient of a disk in a sheet of viscous fluid: numerical calculation. Physica 108A (1981) 598-604.
[16] F.W. Wiegel. Ref. I-10, pg. 135-150.
[17] M. Buas. A theoretical study of membrane diffusion and lymphocyte patching. Ph.D. Thesis, University of Maryland, 1977, unpublished.
[18] F.W. Wiegel and J.R. Heringa. Diffusion coefficient of a protein in a fluid membrane: numerical calculation. Can. J. Phys. 63 (1985) 44-45.
[19] G.I. Bell and A.S. Perelson. Workshop on physical aspects of cellular recognition and response. Aspen Center for Physics. Unpublished report, T-10 Division, Los Alamos National Laboratory, 1981.
[20] M. Bloom. Squishy proteins in fluid membranes. Can. J. Phys. 57 (1979) 2227-2230.
[21] E.L. Elson and J.A. Reidler. Analysis of cell surface interactions by measurements of lateral mobility. J. Supramol. Struct. 6 (1979) 215-228.
[22] J.C. Owicki and H.M. McConnell. Lateral diffusion in inhomogeneous membranes: model membranes containing cholesterol. Biophys. J. 30 (1980) 383-398.
[23] B.A. Smith, W.R. Clark and H.M. McConnell. Anisotropic molecular motion on cell surfaces. Proc. Natl. Acad. Sci. USA 76 (1979) 5641-5644.
[24] A.M. Dykhne. Conductivity of a two-dimensional two-phase system. Zh. Eksp. Teor. Fiz. 59 (1970) 110-115; Sov. Phys. JETP 32 (1970) 63-65.
[25] M.W.M. Willemse and W.J. Caspers. Electrical conductivity of polycrystalline materials. J. Math. Phys. 20 (1979) 1824-1831.[26] M.S. Bretcher. Endocytosis: relation to capping and cell locomotion. Science 224 (1984) 681-686.
[27] F.W. Wiegel. Hydrodynamics of a permeable patch in the fluid membrane. J. Theor. Biol. 77 (1979) 189-193.
[28] B. Goldstein, C. Wofsy and H. Echavarria-Heras. The effect of membrane flow on the capture of receptors by coated pits. Biophys. J. 53 (1988) 405-414.
[29] B. Goldstein and F.W. Wiegel. The distribution of cell surface proteins on spreading cells: comparison of theory with experiment. Biophys. J. 53 (1988) 175-184.
[30] F.W. Wiegel and B. Goldstein. Cap formation by proteins on the cell membrane: excluded volume effects. Mod. Phys. Lett. B2 (1988) 857-859.

VII. EXCLUDED VOLUME EFFECTS IN THE DIFFUSION OF MEMBRANE PROTEINS

1. The kinetic equation

In section II.3 we developed a theory which enables one to calculate the effects of excluded volume on the *equilibrium* distribution of cell membrane proteins. In various situations (like photobleaching recovery experiments) the *kinetics* plays a role. It is the aim of the present chapter to describe a theory which enables one to analyze the effects of excluded volume on the kinetics of proteins which diffuse laterally in the cell membrane, and to apply this theory to some experiments of current interest. We shall also study the case of diffusion in a three dimensional space.

In order to do this we propose two generalizations of the usual time-dependent diffusion equation:

(i) Use an effective, concentration dependent, diffusion constant D(c) to simulate the effects of steric repulsion. It will turn out that this is equivalent to working with the usual diffusion constant D_0 plus an effective steric force field acting on the proteins.

(ii) Use two additional terms which simulate the effects of the sticking of proteins into pockets in which they are effectively surrounded, and hence immobilized, by other objects.

The justification of the proposed kinetic equation is threefold:

(a) When applied to equilibrium the equation gives the correct thermal distribution of the proteins over the cell membrane, including the effects of their steric hindrance, as calculated in [1].

(b) The theory predicts that the <u>experimentally</u> <u>observed</u> diffusion constant decreases sharply with increasing protein concentration.

(c) We can predict the time development of the relaxation towards equilibrium in some experiments.

The ordinary diffusion equation for the concentration c of membrane proteins (number per unit membrane area), which was the subject of chapter VI, can be written as

$$\frac{\partial c}{\partial t} = - \operatorname{div} \vec{\jmath} \tag{1.1}$$

where the current density vector has the special form

$$\vec{\jmath} = - D_T' \, \vec{\nabla} c + \frac{c}{f_T'} \, \vec{F}_{ext} \, , \quad \text{(no steric hindrance)} \, . \tag{1.2}$$

Here D_T' is the diffusion constant, f_T' the friction constant and $\vec{F}_{ext}(\vec{r})$ the external force on a protein. In this chapter we shall restrict ourselves to the case in which all proteins block the same effective area a^2. First, consider the case in which only one type of protein is present.

We suggest that in the presence of steric hindrance one can still use an equation of the form (1.1), but with a current density of the form

$$\vec{\jmath} = -D(c) \, \vec{\nabla} c + \frac{c}{f_T'} \, \vec{F}_{ext} \, , \tag{1.3}$$

where the "effective" lateral diffusion constant $D(c)$ is a function of the protein concentration which we are going to choose in such a way that the equilibrium distribution has the correct form, i.e. the form of eq. (II.3.10)

$$c(\vec{r}) = a^{-2} \ \{1 + e^{+\beta\phi(\vec{r})-\mu}\}^{-1} \ . \qquad \text{(equilibrium)} \ . \qquad (1.4)$$

Here ϕ is the potential of the external force

$$\vec{F}_{ext} = -\vec{\nabla}\phi \ , \qquad (1.5)$$

μ is a constant to be determined later, and $\beta = (k_B T)^{-1}$.

In order to calculate the equilibrium distribution $c(\vec{r})$ from eqs. (1.1-3) one notes that in the case of thermal equilibrium $\vec{J}$ has to vanish everywhere on the membrane, so

$$-D(c)\vec{\nabla}c - \frac{c}{f_T'} \ \vec{\nabla}\phi = 0 \qquad (1.6)$$

everywhere. Dividing by c this can also be written in the form

$$\vec{\nabla} \left\{ \frac{\phi}{f_T'} + \int^{c} \frac{D(c')}{c'} \ dc' \right\} = 0 \ . \qquad (1.7)$$

Hence the quantity within the curly brackets has to be a constant and we find

$$\phi = \text{(constant)} - f_T' \int^{c} \frac{D(c')}{c'} \ dc' \ . \qquad (1.8)$$

This relation has to be identical to the distribution (1.4), which was derived in chapter II from equilibrium statistical physics, and which can be rewritten in the form

$$\phi = k_B T\mu + k_B T \ \ell n \ \frac{1-a^2 c}{a^2 c} \ . \qquad (1.9)$$

It is straightforward to verify that (1.8) and (1.9) are identical if and only if

$$D(c) = \frac{D_T'}{1 - a^2 c} \ , \qquad (1.10)$$

where we used the Einstein relation

$$D_T' \ f_T' = k_B T \ . \qquad (1.11)$$

For the record only we note that the constant in eq. (1.8) has to be equal to (constant) = $k_B T\mu$. Note that the effective diffusion constant (1.10) is independent of the geometry of the cell and does not depend on the external force field but only on the local concentration of the proteins.

To summarize, we have obtained a kinetic equation which follows by combination of eqs. (1.1), (1.3) and (1.10)

$$\frac{\partial c}{\partial t} = + \vec{\nabla} \cdot \left\{ \frac{D_T'}{1 - a^2 c} \ \vec{\nabla}c - \frac{c}{f_T'} \ \vec{F}_{ext} \right\} \qquad (1.12)$$

This equation can be rewritten in the more suggestive form

$$\frac{\partial c}{\partial t} = \vec{\nabla} \cdot \left\{ D'_T \vec{\nabla} c - \frac{c}{f_T} \vec{F}_{steric} - \frac{c}{f_T} \vec{F}_{ext} \right\}$$ (1.13a)

where the term

$$\vec{F}_{steric} = -k_B T \frac{a^2}{1-a^2 c} \vec{\nabla} c$$ (1.13b)

is an effective force due to steric repulsion. Note that this entropic force has all the properties one would intuitively desire: (a) it has the direction of $-\vec{\nabla}c$; (b) it is a local quantity, i.e. it is independent of geometry and of $\vec{F}_{ext}$; (c) it increases with a for constant protein concentrations; (d) it increases with temperature.

2. Generalizations to many species and to sticking

In order to describe some experiments one needs various generalizations of eq. 1.13, which we shall discuss in this section. First, we consider the case in which two protein species diffuse in the membrane (the generalization of this formalism to three or more species is straightforward). Let them be characterized by the same value of the parameter a^2, but be acted on by a different external force $F_{ext}^{(i)}(\vec{r})$ where i = 1,2 labels the two species. This situation applies to a cell with charged- and uncharged protein populations brought into an external electric field. In this case the steric force will depend on the total protein concentration.

$$c = c_1 + c_2$$ (2.1)

and not on the separate concentrations c_1, c_2. Hence the steric force now reads

$$\vec{F}_{steric} = -k_B T \frac{a^2}{1-a^2(c_1+c_2)} \vec{\nabla} (c_1 + c_2) .$$ (2.2)

In this way one finds that the time-dependence of $c_1(\vec{r},t)$ and $c_2(\vec{r},t)$ must now be solved from the coupled equations

$$\frac{\partial c_i}{\partial t} = - \text{div } \vec{J}_i , \qquad (i = 1,2) ,$$ (2.3a)

$$\vec{J}_i = -D'_T \vec{\nabla} c_i + \frac{c_i}{f_T} \left\{ -k_B T \frac{a^2}{1-a^2(c_1+c_2)} \vec{\nabla} (c_1+c_2) + \vec{F}_{ext}^{(i)} \right\}, \ (i=1,2) .$$ (2.3b)

This set of coupled, non-linear, partial differential equations will usually be too hard to solve analytically, hence a numerical procedure will often be necessary.

The second generalization of eq. 1.13 pertains to the need to include the effects of the "sticking" of proteins to other objects in the membrane, as a result of which they are effectively immobilized. One does not have to specify what are the "other objects" to which the proteins can stick. Instead, one has to divide the whole (single species!) protein population into two group: (a) those proteins that are free to diffuse; let them have concentration $c(\vec{r},t)$ and (b) those proteins that are stuck to the "other objects"; let them have the concentration $c^*(\vec{r},t)$. The number of free proteins which get stuck, per unit of time, per unit of surface area, will be written in the form $k_{+}c$, where k_{+} is a phenomenological constant. In the same way there will be $k_{-}c^*$ proteins that were stuck but become unstuck, per unit of time and area. So with this new effect included the single equation (1.12) has to be replaced by the set

$$\frac{\partial c}{\partial t} = \vec{\nabla} \cdot \left\{ \frac{D_T'}{1 - a^2 c} \vec{\nabla} c - \frac{c}{f_T} \vec{F}_{ext} \right\} - k_{+}c + k_{-}c^* ,$$

(2.4a)

$$\frac{\partial c^*}{\partial t} = k_{+}c - k_{-}c^* ,$$

(2.4b)

provided $c^* \ll c$. The set of eqs. (2.4a,b) form the new phenomenological equations which we propose to describe the kinetics of the diffusion of proteins with an excluded volume in cell membranes which carry objects which can immobilize them temporarily. It is easy to verify that in thermal equilibrium ($\partial c/\partial t = 0$, $\partial c^*/\partial t = 0$) the two extra terms $-k_{+}c + k_{-}c^*$ cancel, so the equilibrium solution of (2.4a,b) is still given by eq. 1.4, as required. We now turn to the description of some specific experimental situations.

3. Capture of membrane proteins by a single receptor

As a simple example of the formalism developed in section 1 we consider a single circular receptor, of radius s, which is located in a infinite plane membrane. The concentration of membrane proteins is kept equal to c_0 for $r = R$, where r denotes the radial distance to the center of the receptor. When a protein touches the receptor it is absorbed instantaneously. What is the inward flux (Q) of proteins in the stationary state?

Because of the circular symmetry of this geometry around the center of the receptor the current density must have the form

$$j(r) = - \frac{Q}{2\pi r} ,$$

(3.1)

where the minus sign indicated the fact that the protein current density points towards the receptor. Using for the current the expression (1.3) with $\vec{F}_{ext} = 0$ and D(c) given by (1.10) the last equation reads

$$\frac{D_T'}{1 - a^2 c} \frac{dc}{dr} = \frac{Q}{2\pi r} .$$

(3.2)

This must be solved under the boundary conditions $c(s) = 0$, $c(R) = c_0$. The solution which vanishes for $r = s$ is

$$a^2 c(r) = 1 - \left[\frac{s}{r} \right]^{\frac{a^2 Q}{2\pi D_T'}} ,$$

(3.3)

for any value of Q. Keeping c fixed at the value c_0 for $r = R$ one finds that the receptor captures membrane proteins at a rate

$$Q = \frac{2\pi D_T'}{a^2} \frac{\ell n \ (1 - a^2 c_0)}{\ell n \ (s/R)} .$$

(3.4)

The usual result, in which the effect of the excluded volume of the proteins is neglected, amounts to replacing the Taylor series of the logarithm,

$$\ell n \ (1-a^2c_0) = - \ a^2c_0 - \frac{1}{2} \ (a^2c_0)^2 - \ \dots \ , \tag{3.5}$$

by its first term, giving

$$Q_0 = \frac{2\pi D'_T c_0}{\ell n \ (R/s)} \ . \tag{3.6}$$

Comparison of the second and first term on the right hand side in eq. 3.5 shows that using (3.6) instead of (3.4) underestimates the capture rate by an amount which is a fraction $\frac{1}{2} a^2c_0$ of the estimated capture rate, or $(\frac{1}{2})$ times the fraction of the area which is occupied by proteins.

4. Capture of proteins by a screened coated pit

As a second application, this time of the two-species formalism developed in section 2, we consider the effect of membrane flow on the capture of membrane proteins by a coated pit. We consider the stationary state only. This situation was recently studied in much detail by Goldstein, Wofsy and Echavarría-Heras [VI-28] to whose paper we refer for background information. In the model discussed in this paper the coated pit pulls membrane in at a constant rate; this is equivalent to a membrane-flow field with a radial velocity

$$v(r) = - \frac{\beta}{r} \tag{4.1}$$

which points towards the center of the coated pit. Per unit of time an area $2\pi\beta$ is "ingested" by the coated pit. Of course, due to friction this flow field can as well be described by an external force

$$F_{ext}(r) = - \frac{f'_T \beta}{r} \ ; \tag{4.2}$$

this notation will be used in the following pages.

Now, in most cases there are - roughly speaking - two types of proteins present in the membrane. Species 1, with concentration c_1, will be absorbed by the coated pit at a constant rate Q; species 2 cannot get absorbed by the pit and will form a protective "halo" around it, through which proteins of species 1 have to diffuse in order to get caught. This is just the situation to which eqs. 2.3a,b apply, with $j_1 = - \frac{Q}{2\pi r}$, $j_2 = 0$, $F_{ext}^{(1)} = F_{ext}^{(2)} = - f'_T \beta/r$. Hence one has to solve the set

$$-D'_T \frac{dc_1}{dr} - D'_T \frac{a^2 c_1}{1-a^2(c_1+c_2)} \frac{d}{dr} (c_1+c_2) - \frac{\beta}{r} c_1 = - \frac{Q}{2\pi r} \ , \tag{4.3a}$$

$$-D'_T \frac{dc_2}{dr} - D'_T \frac{a^2 c_2}{1-a^2(c_1+c_2)} \frac{d}{dr} (c_1+c_2) - \frac{\beta}{r} c_2 = 0 \ , \tag{4.3b}$$

subject to certain boundary conditions which will be specified later.

This set of equations can be solved in a straightforward way by first adding them. The total protein concentration

$$c(r) = c_1(r) + c_2(r) \tag{4.4}$$

is the solution of

$$-D_T' \frac{dc}{dr} - D_T' \frac{a^2 c}{1-a^2 c} \frac{dc}{dr} - \frac{\beta}{r} c = -\frac{Q}{2\pi r} . \tag{4.5}$$

This can also be rewritten in the form

$$\frac{D_T'}{a^2} \frac{d}{dr} \ell n (1-a^2 c) - \frac{\beta}{r} c = -\frac{Q}{2\pi r} . \tag{4.6}$$

The general solution can be written as

$$c(r) = \frac{Q}{2\pi \beta} + g(r) , \tag{4.7}$$

where $g(r)$ must be solved from

$$\frac{D_T'}{a^2} \frac{d}{dr} \ell n \left[1 - \frac{a^2 Q}{2\pi \beta} - a^2 g \right] = \frac{\beta}{r} g . \tag{4.8}$$

It is straightforward to verify by substituation that the general solution is

$$g(r) = \left[1 - \frac{a^2 Q}{2\pi \beta} \right] \left\{ a^2 + K r^{\frac{\beta}{D_T'} \left[1 - \frac{a Q}{2\pi \beta} \right]} \right\}^{-1} , \tag{4.9}$$

where K is a positive constant. Note that (4.7) and (4.9) determine the total protein concentration in terms of two unknown positive constants Q and K.

The experiment might, for example, be set up in such a way that the concentration c_1 is fixed at $c_{1,\infty}$ at very large distances from the coated pit and that a total of N proteins of type 2 are present. Hence the boundary condition for their total concentration reads

$$\lim_{r \to \infty} c(r) = c_{1,\infty} . \tag{4.10}$$

Now, eq. 4.9 shows that $g(r)$ always approaches 0 for $r \to \infty$ and hence (4.7) gives

$$Q = 2\pi \beta c_{1,\infty} . \tag{4.11}$$

It is perhaps remakable that in this experiment the flux of type 1 proteins does not depend on their diffusion coefficient D_T'.

The value of the diffusion coefficient D_T' does show up in the separate concentration profiles of the two species. For example, $c_2(r)$ follows from (4.3b) where the steric hindrance term is given by

$$- \frac{a^2}{1-a^2(c_1+c_2)} \frac{d}{dr} (c_1 + c_2) = \frac{d}{dr} \ell n (1-a^2 c) = \frac{a^2}{D_T'} \frac{\beta}{r} g(r) , \tag{4.12}$$

where (4.6) and (4.7) were used. Substitution of the last equation into (4.3) gives

$$-D_T' \frac{dc_1}{dr} + \frac{a^2 \beta g(r)}{r} c_1 - \frac{\beta}{r} c_1 = -\frac{Q}{2\pi r} , \tag{4.13a}$$

$$-D_T' \frac{dc_2}{dr} + \frac{a^2 \beta g(r)}{r} c_2 - \frac{\beta}{r} c_2 = 0 . \qquad (4.13b)$$

The solution of (4.13b) is

$$c_2(r) = \frac{K'}{K \ r^{\beta/D_T'} + a^2 \ r^{a^2 Q/2\pi D_T'}} , \qquad (4.14)$$

where K' denotes another positive constant. Combination of the last equation with (4.7) gives

$$c_1(r) = \frac{Q}{2\pi\beta} + \frac{1 - K' \ r^{-a^2 Q/2\pi D_T'}}{a^2 + K \ r^{\beta/D_T' - a^2 Q/2\pi D_T'}} . \qquad (4.15)$$

For the record only we also note that the two constants K and K' can be determined in the following way. As the coated pit is a perfect absorber for type 1 proteins their concentration should vanish at the edge of the pit. If s denotes the radius of the pit this gives the boundary condition

$$c_1(s) = 0 , \qquad (4.16)$$

which enables one to express K' in terms of K

$$K' = s^{a^2 \beta c_{1,\infty}/D_T'} + c_{1,\infty} (a^2 \ s^{a^2 \beta c_{1,\infty}/D_T'} + K \ s^{\beta/D_T'}) . \qquad (4.17)$$

The value of K follows from the requirement that the total number of type 2 proteins equals N. This gives

$$2\pi \int_0^\infty r \ c_2(r) \ dr = N , \qquad (4.18)$$

which, after substitution of (4.14) and (4.17) and an appropriate scaling of the variable of integration leads to a transcendental equation for K.

The main results of this section are eq. 4.11 for the flux of type 1 proteins into the coated pit and eqs. (4.14, 15) for the concentration profiles. These explicit expressions show that in the stationary state the concentration of the type 2 proteins tends to zero for $r \to \infty$. The type 2 proteins form a protective "halo" around the coated pit because they are swept towards the pit by the combined effects of the membrane flow and the steric interactions with the other proteins (both type 1 and type 2).

5. Ligand diffusion in three dimensions

It should be clear how the formalism of the previous four sections (as well as of II-3) can be generalized to the diffusion of ligands in a three dimensional space. If each protein blocks an effective volume a^3 the equations for a three dimensional diffusion problem follow from those for a two dimensional diffusion problem by replacing

$$a^2 \to a^3 ,$$

$$D'_T \rightarrow D_T , \tag{5.1}$$

$$f'_T \rightarrow f_T .$$

As an example consider the corrections, due to excluded volume, to the problem discussed in chapters III and IV: a sphere of radius s absorbs all ligands which touch its surface anywhere; what is the flux (Q) of ligands in the stationary state? Because of the spherical symmetry of this geometry around the center of the sphere the magnitude of the ligand current density at radial distance r must have the form

$$j(r) = - \frac{Q}{4\pi r^2} . \tag{5.2}$$

Now, for a three dimensional problem (1.3) and (1.10), in the absence of external forces, generalize to

$$\vec{J}(r) = - \frac{D_T}{1 - a^3 c} \vec{\nabla} c . \tag{5.3}$$

Hence the concentration profile can be solved from

$$\frac{-a^3}{1-a^3 c} \frac{dc}{dr} = - \frac{a^3 Q}{4\pi D_T r^2} , \tag{5.4}$$

subject to the boundary conditions $c(s) = 0$, $c(\infty) = c_0$. The solution is

$$\ell n\, (1-a^3 c) = \frac{a^3 Q}{4\pi D_T r} + (\text{constant}) . \tag{5.5}$$

Taking the limit $r \rightarrow \infty$ one finds that the constant equals $\ell n(1 -a^3 c_0)$. On the other hand, setting $r = s$, $c = 0$, one finds

$$0 = \frac{a^3 Q}{4\pi D_T s} + \ell n\, (1-a^3 c_0) , \tag{5.6}$$

hence the flux is given by

$$Q = 4\pi D_T s \cdot \frac{1}{a^3} \ell n \left[\frac{1}{1-a^3 c_0} \right] . \tag{5.7}$$

Of course, for $a^3 c_0 \ll 1$ this equals $4\pi D_T s c_0$, in agreement with eq. (III.2.5) where the flux for *half* a sphere is given.

References to chapter VII

1. B. Goldstein and F.W. Wiegel, in preparation.

VIII. THEORY OF TWO-STAGE CHEMORECEPTION

The central theme of the previous two chapters was the diffusion of proteins in the cell membrane. In this chapter we are going to use some of that work to study two-stage chemoreception, which is related to the ability of most cells to bind certain ligands nonspecifically, i.e. many ligands can bind weakly to the nonreceptor portion of the cell surface as well as specifically to appropriate receptors. Consequently, ligands may bind nonspecifically and then diffuse in the plane of the membrane until they encounter a receptor molecule. Such binding paths are often referred to as non-specific. These paths will be in competition with specific paths that involve binding directly from solution; in general both types of paths will contribute to the rate with which the cell captures ligands. In this short chapter we develop the theory of two-stage chemoreception for the standard model of chapter IV, following some work by Wiegel and DeLisi [1].

The first attempt to model two-stage chemoreception is due to Adam and Delbrück ([I-24], also cf. [I-25] and [I-34]). They used a cylindrical geometry and did not reach a definite conclusion. Yet the basic idea is clearly expressed: the ligand is led to the binding site on the cell by a process of random search in which the dimensionality of the space in which the random walk proceeds is decreased in steps. First the ligand performs diffusion in three-dimensional space until it hits a cell membrane, next it diffuses laterally till it hits the binding site.

Before we discuss the details of our analysis of two-stage chemoreception we would like to point out the possibility that many-stage chemoreception might be realized in nature. For example, many cells carry glycoproteins in their outer membranes. These polymers have long, flexible tails which extend into the extracellular medium and which might actually be involved in facilitating chemoreception. In this case we should speak of three-stage chemoreception: (a) the ligand diffuses through space until it hits the tail of a glycoprotein; (b) it diffuses along this polymer until it hits the cell membrane; (c) it diffuses laterally in the membrane until it hits the receptor. At the time of writing no theory exists for chemoreception in which three-stage capture plays a role. Three-stage capture has some features in common with the association of a repressor to the corresponding operator on the DNA molecule, which process has been studied in considerable detail by Berg and Blomberg [2,3]. It should, therefore, be possible to develop a theory of three-stage chemoreception, but this is left for the future.

We now return to our study of two-stage chemoreception. In order to derive an expression for the rate of ligand capture by a spherical cell in the presence of an external field, we remind the reader of the expression (IV.2.7)

$$c(r) = c(\infty)\lambda(r) - B \lambda (r) \int_r^\infty \rho^{-2} \lambda^{-1} (\rho)d\rho , \qquad (1.1)$$

$$\lambda(r) = \exp \{-\phi(r)/k_B T\} , \qquad (1.2)$$

for the ligand concentration in the space around the cell. The magnitude of the ligand current density at the cell surface $j_N = D_T (\frac{dc}{dr})_{r=R} \frac{1}{1} F(R)c(R)$ is now the sum of two terms

$$j_N = j_N^{(1)} + j_N^{(2)} \; ; \tag{1.3}$$

here $j_N^{(1)}$ is the direct current density into the binding sites of the receptor molecules (cf. eq. IV.1.9)

$$j_N^{(1)} = \alpha \, v \, D_T \, s \, c(R), \tag{1.4}$$

and $j_N^{(2)}$ is the indirect current density due to adsorbed ligands.

The calculation of the latter quantity forces us to adopt a model for the adsorbing properties of the cell membrane, which we choose as follows. Represent the membrane by a square potential well of depth -E < 0 and a thickness d which is approximately equal to the width of the shell to which a bound ligand is constrained. If the volume concentration of ligand just outside the membrane equals c(R) the surface concentration (number of adsorbed ligands per unit area) will be given by the Boltzmann factor

$$n = d \, c(R) \, \exp \, (E/k_B T) \tag{1.5}$$

because close to the membrane adsorbed- and free ligands will be approximately in thermal equilibrium with each other. One can now write

$$j_N^{(2)} = \zeta \, d \, c(R) \, \exp \, (E/k_B T) \; , \tag{1.6}$$

where the value of the propertionality constant ζ will be calculated shortly. Combination of (1.3-6) with the analog of (IV.2.4) gives

$$B = c(\infty) \left\{ \frac{\alpha}{4\pi} \, Ns + \zeta \, R^2 \, \frac{d}{D_T} \, \exp \, (E/k_B T) \right\} \lambda(R) \cdot$$

$$\cdot \left[1 + \left\{ \frac{\alpha}{4\pi} \, Ns + \zeta \, R^2 \, \frac{d}{D_T} \, \exp \, (E/k_B T) \right\} \lambda(R) \int_R^\infty \rho^{-2} \, \lambda^{-1}(\rho) \, d\rho \right]^{-1}. \tag{1.7}$$

Using once more the analog of (IV.2.4), the total flux J_N of ligands into the cell is found to equal

$$J_N = 4 \, \pi \, D_T B \; . \tag{1.8}$$

In order to complete the calculation we need an expression for the parameter ζ.

Consider a spherical cell of radius R, which carries N circular receptors uniformly distributed over the surface. Ligands diffuse laterally in the membrane with a lateral diffusion coefficient D_T'. Moreover, there is a constant flux (q_0) of ligands into the membrane; this flux equals the number of ligands that hit a unit area of the membrane minus the number of ligands that "evaporate" from that area, per unit of time. There are essentially two ways to describe the surface concentration n of ligands in the stationary state.

The first method, followed by all previous authors, amounts to trying to solve the two-dimensional diffusion equation

$$\frac{\partial c'}{\partial t} = D_T' \, \Delta \, c' + q_0 = 0 \tag{1.9}$$

where c' denotes the number of ligands which are adsorbed to the membrane, per unit area. Here Δ denotes the Laplacian in two dimensions. The solution of this equation is subject to the boundary condition

$$c = 0 \text{ on all binding sites.} \tag{1.10}$$

Actually, the complicated nature of the boundary conditions (1.10) makes an analytic solution of (1.9-10) prohibitive. (The results of a numerical solution are discussed in appendix B of ref. [I-34]. Also note that this model is mathematically related to the quantized version of Sinai's billiard, which was recently studied by Berry [4].) Because of this complication, most authors replace the actual boundary condition by the much simpler, but somewhat arbitrary, condition that the normal derivative of c' vanishes everywhere on a circle around each receptor with a radius equal to one half the average distance between receptors.

The second method, which we shall follow in this chapter, uses a coarse-grained description of the type common in the theory of fluid flow in porous media, electromagnetic fields in matter, etc. One defines the coarse-grained surface concentration C' as the average of the surface concentration c' over an area A which is large enough that many receptors are located inside A and small enough that the coarse-grained density C is practically constant within A. The local time variation $\partial C/\partial t$ of this coarse-grained concentration will be caused by: (a) Diffusion, which leads to a term $D_T'\Delta C'$; (b) The constant source density q_0; (c) Absorption of ligands by receptors; this absorption leads to a term $-\zeta C'$. Hence, the stationary state has to be solved from

$$\frac{\partial C'}{\partial t} = D_T' \, \Delta \, C' - \zeta C' + q_0 = 0 \; . \tag{1.11}$$

The solution is

$$C' = C_0' \equiv \frac{q_0}{\zeta} \; . \tag{1.12}$$

The unknown constant ζ can be calculated if one notes that $\zeta \, C_0'/\nu$ by definition equals the number of ligands which are absorbed by a single receptor if the concentration approaches C_0' at a large distance (r) from this receptor. The solution of (1.11) which vanishes for $r \downarrow s$ and which approaches C_0 for $r \to \infty$ is found to equal

$$C'(r) = C_0' \left\{ 1 - \frac{K_0(r \sqrt{\zeta/D_T'})}{K_0(s \sqrt{\zeta/D_T'})} \right\} , \tag{1.13}$$

where the K_n denote the modified Bessel functions. The total lateral flux J_1 into this receptor site is found to be

$$J_1 = 2\pi s D_T' \left| \frac{dC'}{dr} \right|_{r=s} = 2\pi s \sqrt{\zeta D_T'} \; \frac{K_1(s \sqrt{\zeta/D_T'})}{K_0(s \sqrt{\zeta/D_T'})} \, C_0' \; . \tag{1.14}$$

As this should equal $\frac{\zeta}{v} C_0'$ we find the self-consistency condition

$$\phi(\xi) \equiv \xi \frac{K_0(\xi)}{K_1(\xi)} = 2\pi v s^2 \tag{1.15}$$

where

$$\xi = s \sqrt{\zeta/D_T'} . \tag{1.16}$$

This condition implies that ξ^2 is a function $\xi^2(2\pi v s^2)$ of the variable $2\pi v s^2$ only, and hence the parameter ζ is determined by

$$\zeta = \frac{D_T'}{s^2} \xi^2 (2\pi v s^2) . \tag{1.17}$$

The dimensionless parameter $2\pi v s^2$ is of order of the fraction of the cell surface which is occupied by binding sites; this number is typically of order 10^{-3} and hence $\ll 1$. For $\xi \ll 1$ one can approximate (1.15) by $\phi(\xi) \cong \xi^2 |\ell n \xi|$. Therefore, in realistic cases ξ will be small as compared to unity and approximately given by

$$\xi \cong \left\{ \frac{4\pi v s^2}{|\ell n (2\pi v s^2)|} \right\}^{1/2} , \qquad (2\pi v s^2 \ll 1) . \tag{1.18}$$

Combination of (1.17) with (1.18) gives an expression for the parameter ζ in terms of D_T', s^2 and $2\pi v s^2$, which was needed to complete the calculation of the total ligand flux into the cell in the case in which both one-stage and two-stage capture occurs.

In the absence of attractive forces between ligands and cell, the rate of ligand capture by circular receptors equals

$$J_N = 4 \pi R D_T c(\infty) \frac{Ns + \pi R^2 \zeta \frac{d}{D_T} exp (E/k_B T)}{Ns + \pi R + \pi R^2 \zeta \frac{d}{D_T} exp (E/k_B T)} . \tag{1.19}$$

Two-stage capture is switched off by taking the limit $D_T'/D_T \to 0$, in which case the last expression indeed reduces to eq. (IV.3.1) for one-stage chemoreception in the absence of attractive forces.

In the case of an electrostatic attraction, defined by eqs. (IV.3.3,5) the rate of ligand capture by receptors with circular binding sites is found to be given by

$$J_N = 4 \pi R D_T c(\infty) \frac{\{Ns + \pi R^2 \zeta \frac{d}{D_T} exp (E/k_B T)\} e^{\delta/R}}{\pi R + \{Ns + \pi R^2 \zeta \frac{d}{D_T} exp (E/k_B T)\}\frac{R}{\delta}(e^{\delta/R}-1)} \tag{1.20}$$

which reduces to (IV.3.4) when two-stage capture is switched off.

By way of illustration consider the following examples. A cell is involved in chemoreception under the following conditions:

(a) No charge; only one-stage capture; infinitely many receptors. The flux is found by taking the limit $N \to \infty$ in (IV.3.1). This gives the saturation value $J_\infty = 4\pi R D_T c(\infty)$.

(b) As case (a), but with finite N. In order to get 50% of the maximum flux one has to choose $N = \pi R/s \approx 3100$ with the estimates of section IV-3, and $J_N = 2\pi R D_T c(\infty)$.

(c) Electrostatic attraction; only one-stage capture; $N = \pi R/s$. For a charge such that $\delta/R = 1$ the flux is twice its value under conditions (b): $J_N = 4\pi R D_T\, c(\infty)$.

(d) No electrostatic attraction, but both one-stage and two-stage capture processes are permitted. Eq. (1.19) shows that the ratio of the contribution of the non-specific to the direct paths enters essentially through the dimensionless parameter

$$\kappa \equiv \frac{\pi R^2 d}{N s^3} \frac{D_T{}'}{D_T} \exp{(E/k_B T)}\; \xi^2 \left(\frac{N s^2}{2 R^2}\right) , \qquad (1.21)$$

where the dependence of ξ on $Ns^2/2R^2$ was denoted explicitly. Now, as Ns is of order R, d of order s and $\xi^2(Ns^2/2R^2)$ of order Ns^2/R^2 one finds that κ will typically be of order $\frac{D_T{}'}{D_T} \exp{(E/k_B T)}$. Typical values of $D_T{}'/D_T$ are in the range 10^2 to 10^3. Hence two-stage capture processes will be as important as one-stage capture processes if $\exp{(E/k_B T)}$ has values in the range 10^2 to 10^3. At the time of writing no experimental values for the binding energy E are available in the literature; even a rough estimate would serve to indicate the (lack of) importance of two-stage capture processes.

References to chapter VIII

[1] F.W. Wiegel and C. DeLisi. Evaluation of reaction rate enhancement by reduction in dimensionality. Am. J. Physiol. 12 (1982) R475-R479
[2] O.G. Berg and C. Blomberg. Association kinetics with coupled diffusional flows: Special application to the Lac repressor-operator system. Biophys. Chem. 4 (1976) 367-381
[3] O.G. Berg and C. Blomberg. Association kinetics with coupled diffusion: An extension to coiled chain macromolecules applied to the Lac repressor-operator system. Biophys. Chem. 7 (1977) 33-39
[4] M.V. Berry. Quantizing a classically ergodic system: Sinai's billiard and the KKR method. Ann. Phys. 131 (1981) 163-216.

IX. CHEMORECEPTION BY A SWIMMING CELL

In many cases of biological interest the cell which is involved in chemoreception is in a state of uniform motion with respect to the surrounding extracellular fluid. This situation would describe a swimming bacterium, for example. If the cell is described by the standard spherical model with N binding sites, as discussed in section IV.2, one can ask for the effect of swimming on the rate of ligand capture. Up till now this question has not been studied theoretically in a fully satisfactory way. It is the aim of this short chapter to formulate the problem as far as possible, to identify the dimensionless parameters which occur in it, and to solve it in some limiting cases.

The problem of chemoreception by a swimming bacterium was first noted by Berg and Purcell [I-34] (also cf. [1]). It should not be confused with the problem of chemoreception by a cell in shear flow, for which a theoretical analysis is lacking altogether, although some elegant experiments by Purcell [2] have clarified the situation.

Before turning to the details of the calculation some general remarks are appropriate. First, it should once more be stressed that our "standard" model is quite realistic in the sense that chemoreception by a swimming bacterium occurs by a finite number of specific receptor sites rather than continuously everywhere on the cell's surface. This latter case, in which the whole cell surface acts as a perfect ligand absorber, has been studied analytically by Acrivos and Taylor [3]; numerical results can be found in [I-34].

Second, it should be noted that for a bacterium that swims through water with a speed $v_0 \approx 15 \times 10^3$ cm s^{-1} the Reynolds number $Rv_0\rho_0/\eta$ is of order 10^3. Hence, just as in section II.1 the Navier-Stokes equation can be linearized and the fluid velocity field is the Stokes flow (cf. eqs. II.1.8,9)

$$v_r = -v_0 \cos \theta (1 - \frac{3R}{2r} + \frac{R^3}{2r^3}) , \tag{1}$$

$$v_\theta = +v_0 \sin \theta (1 - \frac{3R}{4r} - \frac{R^3}{4r^3}) . \tag{2}$$

Third, one should note that the ligand current density is now given by eq. (IV.1.1) without an external force:

$$\vec{j} = -D_T \vec{\nabla} c + c\vec{v} , \tag{3}$$

hence the diffusion equation has the form

$$\frac{\partial c}{\partial t} = D_T \Delta c - \vec{v} \cdot \vec{\nabla} c , \tag{4}$$

provided the flow is incompressible, which is the case for Stokes flow.

The Peclet number P is defined as the ratio between the order of magnitude of the convective term, $\vec{v} \cdot \vec{\nabla} c \approx v_0 c(\infty)/R$, and of the diffusion term $D_T \Delta c \approx D_T c(\infty)/R^2$

$$P \equiv \frac{v_0 R}{D_T} . \tag{5}$$

Using the expression (II.1.12) for the translational diffusion coefficient and substituting typical orders of magnitude for the various parameters one finds

$$P = \frac{6 \pi \eta \ a \ R \ v_0}{k_B T} \approx 17 \ . \tag{6}$$

For $P \ll 1$ the total ligand current will be close to the limiting form (IV.3.1) derived before. In the rest of this section we consider the asymptotic limit of large Peclet numbers, which is typical for various biophysical situations.

For the stationary state equation (4), when transformed to spherical coordinates, becomes

$$D_T \left\{ \frac{\partial^2 c}{\partial r^2} + \frac{2}{r} \frac{\partial c}{\partial r} + (r^2 \sin\theta)^{-1} \frac{\partial}{\partial \theta} \left(\sin \theta \ \frac{\partial c}{\partial \theta} \right) \right\} = v_r \frac{\partial c}{\partial r} + \frac{v_\theta}{r} \frac{\partial c}{\partial r} \ , \tag{7}$$

where v_r and v_θ are given by the formulae (1,2). The various terms in this equation have different orders of magnitude. For a fixed value of r the concentration will drop from the value $c(\infty)$ in the forward direction $\theta = 0$ to a value close to 0 in the backward direction $\theta = \pi$, hence the estimate

$$\frac{1}{r} \frac{\partial c}{\partial \theta} \approx c(\infty)/R \ . \tag{8}$$

A fluid element close to the cell membrane will need a time of the order R/v_0 to flow around the cell. During this time the ligands will diffuse over distances of order $(R D_T/v_0)^{1/2}$, so one finds the estimate

$$\frac{\partial c}{\partial r} \approx c(\infty) \left[\frac{v_0}{R D_T} \right]^{1/2} \ . \tag{9}$$

This shows that for $P \gg 1$ the third term on the left hand side of (7) can be neglected with respect to the second term. In the same way one shows that the second term is negligible with respect to the first, so the convection- diffusion equation simplifies to

$$D_T \frac{\partial^2 c}{\partial r^2} = v_r \frac{\partial c}{\partial r} + \frac{v_\theta}{r} \frac{\partial c}{\partial \theta} \ , \qquad (P \gg 1). \tag{10}$$

Note that in the layer of thickness $(R D_T/v_0)^{1/2}$ in which the ligand concentration is substantially depleted as a result of ligand diffusion and capture, v_θ will be large compared to v_r, so both terms on the right hand side have to be retained.

In the method of Levich [4] one introduces the function

$$\psi(r,\theta) = \frac{1}{2} v_0 \sin^2 \theta \ (r^2 - \frac{3rR}{2} + \frac{R^3}{2r}) \ , \tag{11}$$

which has the property

$$\left(\frac{\partial \psi}{\partial r} \right)_\theta = r \ v_\theta \sin \theta \ , \tag{12}$$

$$\left(\frac{\partial \psi}{\partial \theta} \right)_r = -r^2 v_r \sin \theta \ , \tag{13}$$

and which, therefore, equals minus the stream function for Stokes flow. Writing the ligand concentration as a function $c(\psi,\theta)$ of the independent variables ψ and θ eq. 10 takes the form

$$\frac{\partial c}{\partial \theta} = D_T r^2 \sin^2 \theta \frac{\partial}{\partial \psi} (r\, v_\theta \frac{\partial c}{\partial \psi}) , \tag{14}$$

where r now denotes the function $r(\psi,\theta)$ which is uniquely defined by inverting (11). For $P \gg 1$ the factor r^2 on the right hand side of this equation can be replaced by R^2 and the factor $r\, v_\theta$ by $(3v_0\psi)^{1/2}$, so the previous equation simplifies further to

$$\frac{\partial c}{\partial \theta} = D_T R^2 \sin^2 \theta \frac{\partial}{\partial \psi} \left\{ (3v_0\psi)^{1/2} \frac{\partial c}{\partial \psi} \right\} . \tag{15}$$

A second coordinate transformation pertinent to this problem consists of replacing θ by

$$\tau = \frac{1}{2} D_T R^2 (3v_0)^{1/2} (\theta - \frac{1}{2} \sin 2\theta) , \quad (0 < \theta < \pi) . \tag{16}$$

This transforms (15) into

$$\frac{\partial c}{\partial \tau} = \frac{\partial}{\partial \psi} (\psi^{1/2} \frac{\partial c}{\partial \psi}) . \tag{17}$$

Hence τ, which essentially measures the azimuthal angle from the direction in which the cell swims, plays the role of time and ψ plays the role of the coordinate in a one-dimensional diffusion problem with a ψ-dependent diffusion coefficient $\psi^{1/2}$. The maximum physically meaningful τ-value is

$$\tau_0 = \frac{\pi}{2} D_T R^2 (3v_0)^{1/2} . \tag{18}$$

The boundary condition at infinity on the function $c(\psi,\tau)$ is

$$c(\infty,\tau) = c(\infty) , \qquad (0 < \tau < \tau_0) . \tag{19}$$

We also require the concentration to be equal to $c(\infty)$ on the whole line $\theta = 0$, $R < r < \infty$ in the forward direction; this leads to the initial condition

$$c(\psi,0) = c(\infty), \qquad (0 < \psi < \infty) . \tag{20}$$

Finally, at the surface of the cell one imposes the boundary condition (IV.1.9), with $V = 0$ because of the absence of external forces. Transformation to the ψ,τ coordinates gives the boundary condition

$$c = \varepsilon' \sin \theta \; \psi^{1/2} (\frac{\partial c}{\partial \psi})_\tau , \qquad (\psi = 0, \; 0 < \tau < \tau_0) \tag{21}$$

in the limit $\psi \to 0$; here $\sin \theta$ should be interpreted as a function of τ through (16) and ε' denotes the constant

$$\varepsilon' = \frac{4\pi R^2}{\alpha N s} (3v_0)^{1/2} . \tag{22}$$

The general solution of (8.17) can be expanded in Bessel functions of the first kind and has the form

$$c(\psi,\tau) = c(\infty) + \psi^{1/4} \int_0^\infty [A(\lambda) \, J_{1/3} \, (\tfrac{4}{3} \lambda^{1/2} \, \psi^{3/4}) + B(\lambda) \, J_{-1/3}(\tfrac{4}{3} \lambda^{1/2} \, \psi^{3/4})].$$

$$. \exp(-\lambda\tau)d\lambda \, . \tag{23}$$

The boundary condition (19) shows that the functions $A(\lambda)$ and $B(\lambda)$ vanish for $\lambda < 0$. The initial condition (20) is satisfied provided these functions are related by

$$\int_0^\infty [A(\lambda) \, J_{1/3} \, (\tfrac{4}{3} \lambda^{1/2} \, \psi^{3/4}) + B(\lambda) \, J_{-1/3}(\tfrac{4}{3} \lambda^{1/2} \, \psi^{3/4})]d\lambda = 0, \quad (0<\psi<\infty) \, . \tag{24}$$

The boundary condition (21) becomes

$$c(0,\tau) \equiv c(\infty) + \Gamma^{-1} \, (2/3) \, (2/3)^{-1/3} \int_0^\infty B(\lambda)\lambda^{-1/6} \, e^{-\lambda\tau} \, d\lambda$$

$$= \tfrac{1}{2} \, \varepsilon' \sin \theta \, \Gamma^{-1} \, (4/3) \, (2/3)^{1/3} \int_0^\infty A(\lambda)\lambda^{1/6} \, e^{-\lambda\tau} \, d\lambda, \, (0<\tau<\tau_0). \tag{25}$$

Although the two unknown functions $A(\lambda)$ and $B(\lambda)$ are in principle determined by the last two equations, their explicit evaluation has not yet been possible. These equations show that, as ψ is of order $v_0 R^2$ and $\partial c/\partial \psi$ of order $c(\infty)R^{-3/2} \, D_T^{-1/2} \, v_0^{-1/2}$, the solution will depend not on ε' but on the dimensionless combination

$$\varepsilon = \frac{R}{Ns} \, P^{1/2} \tag{26}$$

of the Peclet number P, which determines the convection-diffusion problem, and the parameter R/Ns which determines chemoreception by a cell at rest.

If $\varepsilon \ll 1$ the right hand sides of (21,25) can approximately be set equal to zero. In this case one can follow the much simpler method of Levich [4] who noticed that both the differential equation (17) and its boundary conditions are invariant under the substitutions

$$\psi = \mu \, \psi' \, , \tag{27a}$$

$$\tau = \mu^{3/2} \, \tau' \, . \tag{27b}$$

This suggests looking for a solution which is a function $c(\eta)$ of the combination

$$\eta \equiv \psi \, \tau^{-2/3} \, , \tag{28}$$

c.f. Dresner [5]. The convection-diffusion equation now becomes an ordinary differential equation

$$\frac{d}{d\eta} \, (\eta^{1/2} \frac{dc}{d\eta}) + \frac{2}{3} \, \eta \, \frac{dc}{d\eta} = 0 \, , \tag{29}$$

with boundary conditions

$$c(\eta = 0) = 0 \; , \qquad c(\eta = \infty) = c(\infty) \; . \tag{30a,b}$$

The solution is

$$c(\eta) = c(\infty) \; \frac{\int_0^{\eta^{1/2}} \exp(-\tfrac{4}{9} z^3) \, dz}{\int_0^{\infty} \exp(-\tfrac{4}{9} z^3) \, dz} \; . \tag{31}$$

The ligand current density is given by

$$j = D_T (3v_0)^{1/2} \sin \theta \; \lim_{\psi \to 0} \psi^{1/2} \left(\frac{\partial c}{\partial \psi}\right)_\tau$$

$$= K \, D_T \, c(\infty) \left(\frac{v_0}{D_T R^2}\right)^{1/3} \frac{\sin \theta}{(\theta - \tfrac{1}{2} \sin 2\theta)^{1/3}} \; , \tag{32}$$

where the numerical constant has the value

$$K = (1/3)^{1/3} \, \Gamma^{-1}(4/3) = 0.7765 \; . \tag{33}$$

Finally, the total ligand flux into the cell is found to equal

$$J = \tfrac{3}{2} \pi^{5/3} \, K \, c(\infty) \, D_T^{2/3} \, R^{4/3} \, v_0^{1/3} = 7.849 \, c(\infty) \, D_T^{2/3} \, R^{4/3} \, v_0^{1/3}, \; (P \gg 1, \varepsilon \ll 1). \tag{34}$$

Comparing this flux with the ligand flux J_∞ into a perfectly absorbing cell at rest the ratio is proportional to the one-third power of the Peclet number ($J/J_\infty = \tfrac{3}{8} \pi^{2/3} \, K \, P^{1/3} = 0.6246 \, P^{1/3}$). Hence swimming is of little help to improve the efficiency of chemoreception, unless the cell swims very fast, which will necessitate a very high rate of energy consumption.

References to chapter IX

[1] E.M. Purcell. Life at low Reynolds numbers. Am. J. Phys. 45 (1977) 3-11.
[2] E.M. Purcell. The effect of fluid motions on the absorption of molecules by suspended particles. J. Fluid Mech. 84 (1978) 551-559.
[3] A. Acrivos and T.D. Taylor. Heat and mass transfer from single spheres in Stokes flow. Phys. Fluids 5 (1962) 387-394.
[4] B.G. Levich. Physicochemical Hydrodynamics (Prentice-Hall, Englewood Cliffs, 1962).
[5] L. Dresner. Similarity Solutions of Nonlinear Partial Differential Equations (Pitman, London, 1983).